T0235848

Discovery DMPK Quick Guide

S. Cyrus Khojasteh • Harvey Wong
Donglu Zhang • Cornelis E.C.A. Hop

Discovery DMPK Quick Guide

Guide to Data Interpretation and Integration

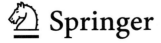 Springer

S. Cyrus Khojasteh
Genentech, Inc.
South San Francisco, CA, USA

Donglu Zhang
Genentech, Inc.
South San Francisco, CA, USA

Harvey Wong
University of British Columbia
Vancouver, BC, Canada

Cornelis E.C.A. Hop
Genentech, Inc.
South San Francisco, CA, USA

Editorial Contact
Carolyn Spence

ISBN 978-3-031-10693-4   ISBN 978-3-031-10691-0   (eBook)
https://doi.org/10.1007/978-3-031-10691-0

This Springer imprint is published by the registered company Springer Nature Switzerland AG
The registered company address is: Gewerbestrasse 11, 6330 Cham, Switzerland

Foreword

Drug discovery is one of the most exciting fields in science today. The profession requires constant learning of emerging areas of research while maintaining dedication, persistence, and innovation. As drug metabolism and pharmacokinetic (DMPK) scientists, we look through the lens of druggability by examining absorption, distribution, metabolism, and excretion (ADME). The ADME sciences have expanded to include the examination of various barriers that prevent a drug from reaching the site of action (target). As the field of DMPK expands, researchers may find it difficult to be knowledgeable in all the different areas involved in their work. This book is an attempt to provide DMPK scientists with a quick reference guide that can answer specific questions in a practical manner, mainly focused on the drug discovery stage.

One of the key aspects of ADME science is understanding the specific liabilities that need to be addressed for each potential drug. This requires understanding the various ADME assay outputs plus the chemistry behind the molecule's behavior. Importantly, advances in *in silico* predictive sciences have allowed for the exploration of ideas prior to the actual synthesis of molecules. Assay cascades are then typically put in place to create focus and a specific sequence of studies during the drug discovery process. Note that sometimes molecules are progressed to different stages of the cascade so that specific properties can be investigated. In addition, the final candidate has to overcome various barriers to reach the intended target. The decision-making process required to single out the final candidate requires a high level of technical expertise plus strategic understanding of the project and experience.

In our first book, *Quick Guide to Drug Metabolism and Pharmacokinetics*, we explored topics such as PK, drug metabolism, and transport. Here, we focus on the application of these concepts during drug discovery, and we provide a template for decision-making during this stage. The information in this book mainly applies to small molecules, but we also touch upon new modalities including covalent inhibitors, macrocyclic peptides, and degraders.

The chapters are organized so that each one can be read independently. You will notice gray boxes that contain remarks and factoids to complement that section. Each section also includes case studies that are relevant to the topic being discussed. You will find the listed case studies at the beginning of each section.

We hope that you will find this book to be a useful reference as you work to discover new and novel medicines.

Thank you,
S. Cyrus Khojasteh, on behalf of all authors

Contents

About the Authors

S. Cyrus Khojasteh is a Senior Director and Senior Principal Scientist and heads the Biotransformation Function in DMPK Department at Genentech (South San Francisco). He leads the ADME efforts of macrocyclic peptides and microbiome efforts. His biotransformation research focuses on the mechanisms of biotransformation in drug discovery and development, from small molecules, antibody drug conjugates, and macrocyclic peptides. Cyrus received his PhD in medicinal chemistry from the University of Washington under the direction of Professor Sidney D. Nelson.

Harvey Wong is Associate Professor of Pharmacokinetics in the Faculty of Pharmaceutical Sciences at the University of British Columbia. He obtained his BSc in pharmacy and PhD in pharmacokinetics and biopharmaceutics from the University of British Columbia (Canada). Harvey's expertise is in pharmacokinetics, and modeling and simulation (translational PK/PD analysis, systems pharmacology, and physiologically based pharmacokinetic modeling). He serves on the editorial boards of *Biopharmaceutics and Drug Disposition*, *Xenobiotica*, and *Clinical and Translational Sciences*.

Donglu Zhang is a Senior Fellow in DMPK at Genentech. He is interested in applying drug metabolism studies in drug design and development of both small molecule drugs, protein degraders, and antibody-drug conjugates (ADC). He received the Sir James Black Award for discovery of and original research on Eliquis from the British Pharmacological Society (2018), and the Ondetti and Cushman Award for invention of mass defect filtering method (MDF) from Bristol-Myers Squibb (2007). He serves on editorial boards of *Drug Metabolism and Disposition* and *Xenobiotica*.

Cornelis E.C.A. Hop is Vice President at Genentech and supervises the DMPK Department. He leads a team of about 85 scientists involved in acquisition and interpretation of ADME data in support of drug discovery and development ranging from early stage research to NDA and beyond. Before that he was a senior director at Pfizer and a senior research fellow at Merck, and he received his PhD from the University of Utrecht (the Netherlands). He has extensive experience in ADME sciences with a particular focus on PK optimization, human PK prediction, biotransformation, bioanalysis, and the use of *in silico* approaches in drug discovery.

Other Contributors

Contributions were made during their time at Genentech, Inc.
Ignacio Aliagas, Senior Scientist
Sungjoon Cho, Scientist
Kevin Johnson, Senior Scientist
Ivy Kekessie, Principal Scientific Researcher
Shuguang Ma, Senior Principal Scientist
Emile Plise, Senior Principal Scientific Researcher
Dian Su, Principal Scientist
Shuai Wang, Senior Scientist
Zhengyin Yan, Senior Principal Scientist

List of Figures

List of Tables

Chapter 1
Goals for DMPK During Drug Optimizations

Contents

Abstract In the discovery stage, one of the key parameters that is optimized is the drug activity towards a specific target (potency). Potency is measurement of a molecule's interaction/modulation of a therapeutic target. What allows conversion of a potent chemical starting point to a final drug/drug candidate during the optimization process is the incorporation of appropriate ADME properties that balance efficacy and toxicity. Here we capture the high-level drug discovery optimization process with an emphasis on optimization of ADME properties.

Keywords Absorption · Distribution · Metabolism · And excretion · Optimization · Strategy · Target candidate profile · Pharmacodynamics · Pharmacokinetics

Abbreviations

ADME	Absorption, distribution, metabolism, and excretion
C_{max}	C_{max} is the highest concentration of a drug in the blood after a given dose
CNS	Central nervous system
DMPK	Drug metabolism and pharmacokinetics
FDA	Food and Drug Administration
GI	Gastrointestinal
hERG	Human Ether-à-go-go-related (a potassium ion channel)

© Springer Nature Switzerland AG 2022
S. C. Khojasteh et al., *Discovery DMPK Quick Guide*,
https://doi.org/10.1007/978-3-031-10691-0_1

IC$_{50}$	Half maximal inhibitory concentration
NME	New molecular entity
PD	Pharmacodynamics
PK	Pharmacokinetics
POC	Proof of concept
R&D	Research and development
TCP	Target candidate profile

1.1   ADME Objectives

Drug discovery and development remains a very challenging endeavor fraught with a very high attrition rate. Even though the number of FDA approvals has gone up, this may be a direct consequence of increased funding in the biopharmaceutical industry. Successful discovery projects frequently necessitate the synthesis of more than 1000 compounds. Unfortunately, most discovery projects never yield a viable development candidate. Preclinical attrition is frequently multi-faceted, but broadly encompasses three major categories:

1. Lack of preclinical proof of concept (POC) showing that modulating the target will result in the desired effect in an animal model. This is a major source of attrition for novel targets, but much less so for fast follow up drugs that attempt to improve the properties of existing drugs.
2. Insurmountable preclinical safety signals. The challenge here is that the exposure resulting in toxicity must be seen in light of the exposure required for efficacy. However, the latter may not be known (yet) and, therefore, a conservative stance is usually adopted, especially for non-oncology projects. Finally, translatability of toxicological findings in rodents and non-rodents to – ultimately – humans is often questionable.
3. The inability to balance desirable properties, such as potency, selectivity, ADME and tolerability in one molecule. Drug hunters are usually quite experienced in finding a needle in a haystack, but in some cases, the driving forces that govern different properties are diametrically opposed. Hence, these targets are sometimes deemed 'undruggable'.

> Nature has raised an enormous barrier to drug development by assigning the drug-metabolizing enzymes to various species in astonishingly diverse amount. So great are these differences that it is often a matter of pure luck that animal experiment lead to clinical useful drug.
> Bernard B. Brodie, Ph.D.

> Bernard Beryl Brodie (1907–1989) is considered to be the founder of modern pharmacology. He was a founder and former chief of the Laboratory of Chemical Pharmacology at the National Heart Institute of the National Institutes of Health in Bethesda, Maryland.

Attrition in development is high as well. It has been shown that attrition in all phases of development – from preclinical development to registration – has gradually increased and in particular in phase 2 due to the inability to achieve pharmacological proof of concept (Pammolli et al. 2011). Consequently, people have called out that trends in drug discovery and development are the opposite of Moore's law, where the number of transistors in an integrated circuit – and hence the number of calculations per second – doubles roughly every two years. Indeed, the number of drugs discovered per billion dollars invested in R & D has been gradually declining. However, positive trends have been are observed in the last 5 to 10 years. The number of drug approvals per year has been increasing gradually with 53 approvals in 2020 by the US Food & Drug Administration (Mullard 2021). Some biopharmaceutical companies have introduced specific strategies to tackle attrition and they appear to be successful. For example, AstraZeneca introduced the 5R principles to increase focus on key attributes that matter in drug discovery and development (Cook et al. 2014) Fig. 1.1.

Implementation of the 5R principles at AstraZeneca resulted in significantly reduced attrition. In particular, the success rate in phase 2 clinical studies increased from 15% to 29% (Morgan et al. 2018). Moreover, attrition due to PK and PK/PD reasons reduced and 76% of the human PK predictions between 2012 and 2016

Right target:
- Strong link between target and disease
- Differentiated efficacy
- Available and predictable biomarkers

Right tissue:
- Adequate bioavailability and tissue exposure
- Definition of PD biomarkers
- Clear understanding of preclinical and clinical PK/PD
- Understanding of drug-drug interactions

Right safety:
- Differentiated and clear safety margin
- Understanding of secondary pharmacology risk
- Understanding of reactive metabolites, genotoxicity, drug-drug interactions
- Understanding of target liability

Right patient:
- Identification of the most responsive patient population
- Definition of risk-benefit for given population

Right commercial potential:
- Differentiated value propositions versus future standard of care
- Focus on market access, payer and provider
- Personalized heath-care strategy, including diagnostics and biomarkers

Fig. 1.1 The 5R principles at AstraZeneca. (Cook et al. 2014)

were within two-fold of the observed clinical exposure. The latter is remarkable because PK and bioavailability were the major source of clinical attrition up to 1991(Kola and Landis 2004). Similarly, Pfizer made significant improvements in its phase 2 attrition by rigorous implementation of their three pillars model, which stipulated that *"for a development candidate to have the potential to elicit the desired pharmacological effect over the necessary period of time, three fundamental elements needed to be demonstrated: exposure at the site of action (Pillar 1); binding to the pharmacological target (Pillar 2); and expression of pharmacological activity from the site of action (Pillar 3)"* (Wu et al. 2021). Before rigorous implementation of this model, it was not always clear if a compound attrited in phase 2 clinical studies because

1. the targeted mechanism simply did not result in the desired human pharmacological response or
2. the exposure was insufficient to result in a human pharmacological response.

If attrition is due to lack of exposure, a backup compound could fix that, but if the compound fails because modulation of the target does not result in the desired pharmacological response in the clinic, termination of the project is essential. These new operating models place increased importance on biomarkers and an understanding of the PK/PD relationship. Finally, the arsenal of molecular modalities is expanding – including covalent inhibitors, (macrocyclic) peptides, degraders, RNA modulators, etc. – and they each have their unique set of challenges. In this book, we will look at the use of ADME principles in the drug discovery process and how these principles need to go hand in hand with optimization of potency, selectivity, tolerability, etc. to find a drug with the right balance of properties and, hence, increased probability of making it all the way to the market place to address high medical need.

ADME Science   ADME science has broad objectives. From the pharmacological angle, the goal is to determine how the drug elicits its desired pharmacological effects, which is defined by the drug's residence time at the site of action (Stromgaard et al. 2016). From the drug perspective, the goal is to identify the effects of the biological system (i.e., the human body) on the drug, from the moment it enters the body to its elimination. The combined ADME and potency properties of a specific molecule allow one to understand the relationships between dose, exposure, and pharmacological activity. This dynamic relationship between drug kinetics and drug effect is described by pharmacokinetics and pharmacodynamics, respectively.

Drug Discovery   One focus of drug discovery is the optimization of ADME properties to best elicit a pharmacological effect while minimizing toxicity (Dörwald 2012). The discovery could be divided into three stages (each company uses different names but the context would be similar). (1) Hit-seeking stage, (2) Lead-seeking stage, and (3) Candidate-seeking stage (Fig. 1.2). At each stage the search area narrows to more specific chemical space. At the end of these stages, a specific molecule is considered ready for clinical development as a new molecular entity (NME).

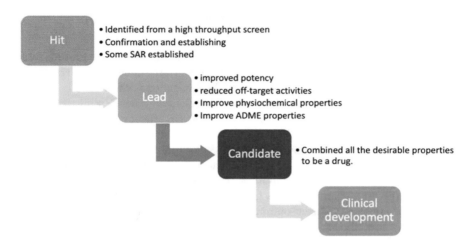

Fig. 1.2 The different stages of drug discovery: the hit-seeking, lead-seeking, and candidate-seeking stages

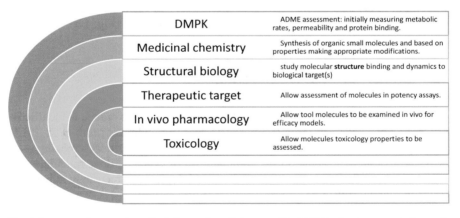

Fig. 1.3 Experts from various disciplines who collaborate with ADME scientists to optimize molecules during drug discovery. Drug metabolism and pharmacokinetics (DMPK) scientists are researchers that examine ADME sciences

1.2 Expertise Needed During Drug Discovery

Several experts are needed to come together to optimize the features of a compound during the discovery stage. They are listed in Fig. 1.3.

The resources needed from each of these scientists will change as the issues that need to be addressed shift during the optimization process. In most cases, the resource needs increase as the project is getting closer to candidate selection. Typically, the earlier assays are fewer with higher capacity, while later on in the process, more definitive assays are conducted to broaden the scope of the assessment.

1.3 Optimization of ADME Properties

Optimization of ADME properties allows for moving chemical space towards more drug-like properties. This requires the identification of the chemical drivers of efficacy, toxicity, and ADME. The overview of the navigation is shown in Fig. 1.4.

Prior to the 1990's, decision-making heavily relied on potency while neglecting *in vitro* ADME assessments, except for *in vivo* PK and efficacy (phenotypic assessment) (Zhang and Surapaneni 2012). The risk of this strategy was that many compounds that proceeded to target-specific screening (potency-focused optimization) were found to be in such chemical space that ADME challenges were inevitable. Moreover, there was no appreciation of the translatability – or lack thereof – of preclinical PK to human PK. Thus, high attrition because of PK and bioavailibity reasons was inevitable. The co-optimization of several parameters, which is usually what occurs now, allows for several properties to be investigated simultaneously in lead molecules. However, note that good judgement is needed to pursue compounds that may be suboptimal in certain areas but still have the potential to be drugs.

Modern drug discovery involves the assessment of many different properties including structural, chemical, and *in vitro* and *in vivo* behaviors (Caldwell and Yan 2014). An understanding of ADME properties allows for a proper evaluation of when a drug can elicit its desired efficacy at the site of action (Fig. 1.5).

1.4 Modern ADME Optimization

Understanding the key stage-specific liability (or liabilities) is crucial at the discovery stage since decisions are made based on ADME liabilities (Smith et al. 2012). Placement of specific assays in the discovery cascade creates critical screening – and hence optimization – points for the compounds. For example, drug candidates can be assessed separately in relation to different biological barriers, thus influencing decision-making (Fig. 1.6).

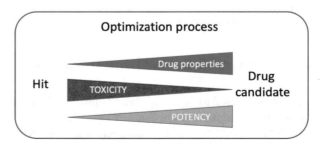

Fig. 1.4 Depiction of the overall optimization pathway during the process of going from hit to candidate

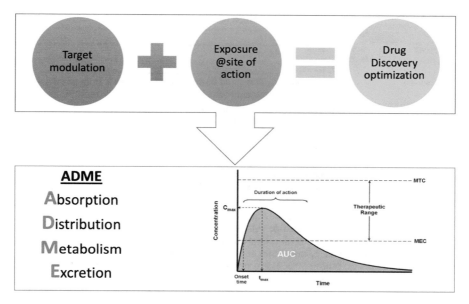

Fig. 1.5 ADME contribution to drug efficacy – assessing absorption (A), distribution (D), metabolism (M), and excretion (E) to determine whether a drug can reach the intended target

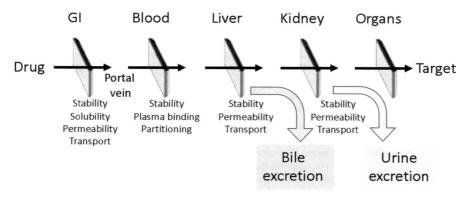

Fig. 1.6 Barriers to reaching the target for orally administered drugs

A document can be put together for each project that defines the desired profile for the ideal candidate. This document is frequently called a target candidate profile (TCP) and allows the project team to aim for specific drug properties within a framework of support for minimal toxicity and suitable efficacy (Table 1.1).

Table 1.1 Desired properties captured in a target candidate profile (TCP)

Properties	Prototype criteria
Biological considerations	Biological evidence
Indications	The indications that could be considered. Feedback from physicians and understanding the competitive landscape for the indications will be very useful. High level questions should be asked, which allow the project team to focus their efforts. For example, what route of administration provides the highest patient compliance
Potency	**Biochemical potency:** $IC_{50} \leq X$ nM **Cell-based potency:** $IC_{50.} \leq X$ nM **Selectivity:** X-fold against selected targets Plasma binding may play a role. So assays may have to be established to consider this parameter
DMPK	Dosing route: Oral, IV, SC, inhalation, others? PK compatible with the desired dosing interval PK properties: Oral absorption >X% in preclinical species at therapeutic doses and above (for safety assessment). X% is typically above 30%. There are times that it is acceptable to have one of the species to be lower in %F, but mechanistic considerations are needed for making sure that it does not translate to humans. Low %F leads to high PK variability CNS permeability: Is this is a desirable property or not? It should be called out
Safety	Considerations depend on the indication and duration **In vivo:** Toxicities that are manageable, monitorable, reversible in rodent / non-rodent; safety margin should be appropriate for the proposed patient population **In vitro:** No mutagenicity (Ames) or clastogenicity (micronucleus) hERG IC_{50} >X-fold over projected human efficacious free-drug C_{max}
In vivo PD/efficacy	Define *in vivo* preclinical disease model (if it exists) Perform *in vivo* studies for determining the dose-dependent effect of target modulation
Pharmaceutical sciences	Projected dose to be <X milligram daily based on preclinical efficacy models to keep pill burden managable
Clinical biomarkers	Clinical biomarkers that are expected to be helpful in patient selection, target engagement or disease improvement. Finding suitable biomarkers could be a game-changer as one enters the clinic and provides confidence in the suitability of the target and/or disease modulation

References

Caldwell GW, Yan Z (2014) Optimization in drug discovery. In: vitro methods (methods in pharmacology and toxicology), 2nd edn ISBN-10: 1493960709

Cook D, Brown D, Alexander R, March R, Morgan P, Satterthwaite G, Pangalos MN (2014) Lessons learned from the fate of AstraZeneca's drug pipeline: a five-dimensional framework. Nat Rev Drug Discov 13(6):419–431

Dörwald FZ (2012) Lead optimization for medicinal chemists: pharmacokinetic properties of functional groups and organic compounds. ISBN: 978-3-527-33226-7

Kola I, Landis J (2004) Can the pharmaceutical industry reduce attrition rates? Nat Rev Drug Discov 3(8):711–715

Morgan P, Dean G, Brown DG et al (2018) Impact of a five-dimensional framework on R&D productivity at AstraZeneca. Nat Rev Drug Discov 17(3):167–181

Mullard A (2021) 2020 FDA drug approvals. Nat Rev Drug Discov 20(2):85–90

Pammolli F, Magazzini L, Riccaboni M (2011) The productivity crisis in pharmaceutical R & D. Nat Rev Drug Discov 10(6):428–438

Smith DA, Allerton C, Kalgutkar AS et al (2012) Pharmacokinetics and metabolism in drug design. In: Methods and principles in medicinal chemistry book 51, 3rd edn. Wiley-VCH

Stromgaard K, Krogsgaard-Larsen P, Madsen U (2016) Textbook of drug design and discovery. CRC Press. ISBN 9781498702782

Wu SS, Fernando K, Allerton C et al (2021) Reviving an R&D pipeline: a step change in the phase II success rate. Drug Discov Today 26(2):308–314

Zhang D, Surapaneni S (eds) (2012) ADME-enabling technologies in drug design and development, 1st edn. Wiley. https://doi.org/10.1002/9781118180778

Chapter 2
Drug Properties

Contents

Abstract Drug discovery remains a complex and iterative process accompanied with a high failure rate. Before compounds enter the clinic, failures can be due to (1) an inability to demonstrate that the target can modulate the disease in a preclinical model, (2) the lack of a therapeutic index to modulate the target safely or (3) the inability to find molecules with the right balance of properties such as potency, selectivity, ADME properties, safety endpoints, etc. Moreover, drug discovery is geting harder because of the pursuit of targets that are deemed 'undruggable'. What makes a target 'undruggable' is usually the lack of a distinct binding pocket that is unique. Two fundamental approaches to drug discovery exist: structure-based design and property-based design. In this chapter we capture the molecular properties that influence and drive drug discovery. In addition, for each class of drugs we captured their distinct properties.

© Springer Nature Switzerland AG 2022   11
S. C. Khojasteh et al., *Discovery DMPK Quick Guide*,
https://doi.org/10.1007/978-3-031-10691-0_2

Keywords Physicochemical properties · Multi-parameter optimization · Drug properties · Therapeutic targets · Pharmacodynamics · Pharmacokinetics · Biopharmaceutics Classification System · Biopharmaceutics Drug Disposition Classification System · Clearance · Covalent inhibitor · Central nervous system · Cytochrome P450 · Extended Clearance Classification System

Abbreviations

5-HMT	5-hydroxymethyl tolterodine
ABT	1-aminobenzotriazole
AI	Artificial intelligence
ALK	Anaplastic lymphoma kinase
AO	Aldehyde oxidase
API	Active pharmaceutical ingredient
ATP	Adenosine triphosphate
BCS	Biopharmaceutics Classification System
BDDCS	Biopharmaceutics Drug Disposition Classification System
BMO	Biomimetic metalloporphyrin oxidation
CI	Covalent inhibitor (also known as covalent modifiers)
CL	Clearance
CNS	Central nervous system
CYP	Cytochrome P450
ECCS	Extended Clearance Classification System
EM	Electron microscopy
FaSSIF	Fasted state simulated intestinal fluid
FeSSIF	Fed state simulated intestinal fluid
FMO	Flavin-containing monooxygenase
GPCR	G protein-coupled receptor
HAT	Hydrogen atom abstraction
HBA	Hydrogen bond accepter
HBD	Hydrogen bond donor
ID	Infectious diseases
IV	Intravenous administration
IVIVC	*in vitro – in vivo* correlation
KIE	Kinetic isotope effect
LipE	Lipophilic efficiency
LLE	Lipophilic ligand efficiency
logD	Distribution coefficient
logP	Partition coefficient
MD	Metabolic diseases
MPO	Multi-parameter optimization
MW	Molecular weight
NAR	Number of aromatic rings

NMR	Nuclear magnetic resonance
NRB	Number of rotatable bonds
NVP	Nevirapine
ONC	Oncology
PDB	Protein data bank
P-gp	P-glycoprotein
PK	Pharmacokinetics
PO	Oral administration
PPi	Protein-protein interaction
PSA	Polar surface area
Ro5	Rule of 5; Lipinski's rule
SET	Topological single electron transfer
TPSA	Topological polar surface area
UGT	Glucuronosyltransferase
V_d	Volume of distribution

Case Studies

Case	Topic	Molecules
2.1	Isosteres to improve solubility.	Tioconazole & fluconazole
2.2	Discovery of macrocycle lorlatinib from crizotinib using structure-based drug design	Lorlatinib from crizotinib
2.3	Use of a prodrug to enhance solubility.	Chloramphenicol, diazepam and their prodrugs
2.4	Use of a prodrug to decrease first pass metabolism	Propranolol and its prodrug
2.5	Use of a prodrug to improve permeability	Amidine-containing molecules and their O-methoxy- and O-ethoxy-amidine analogues
2.6	Use of a prodrug to improve oral bioavailability by uptake transport	Levodopa to dopamine; valacyclovir, valganciclovir and midodrine
2.7	Use of a prodrug to increase chemical stability	Hetacillin and penicillin
2.8	Hydroxyamidine as a prodrug and the involvement of mARC	Upamostat and WX-UK1
2.9	Active metabolites as drugs	Codeine, morphine and morphine-6-glucuronide; amitriptyline and nortriptyline
2.10	Polymorphism of drug metabolizing enzymes can influence drug design	Tamoxifen and endoxifen; tolterodine and fesoterodine
2.11	Metabolites with lower toxicity	Hydroxyzine, cetirizine and levocetirizine; terfenadine and fexofenadine

2.1 Impact of Physicochemical Properties on ADME Parameters

2.1.1 Structure-Based Design

Structure-based design hinges on the availability of the crystal structure of either the native protein or (preferably) the protein with an active molecule in the binding pocket (a co-crystal). This approach has been successfully applied to many types of targets and it has been particularly successful for the discovery of many kinase inhibitors. In early 2021, the protein data bank (PDB) contained more than 175,000 protein structures and the majority were obtained by X-ray crystallography and to a lesser extent nuclear magnetic resonance (NMR). X-ray crystallography requires high quality crystals of a finite size. However, generation of those crystals and co-crystals can be laborious or impossible, in particular for membrane targets such as ion channels, because of the difficulty of the protein to adopt a stable, crystallizable structure. More recently, cryogenic electron microscopy (cryo-EM) has been deployed and, in contrast to x-ray crystallography, it requires only minute crystals. However, the equipment required for cryo-EM is expensive and the spatial resolution is frequently still less than that obtained with x-ray crystallography. However, the cryo-EM technology is progressing rapidly and results have been generated that cannot be obtained with the conventional techniques.

The availability of the crystal structure of the protein target with an active molecule in its binding pocket provides a three-dimensional picture of the interactions required for binding to the target and that information can be used to design molecules that may make better and more specific interactions with the protein target and, hence, results in improved potentcy. An example is presented in Fig. 2.1. It shows the crystal structure of a competitive inhibitor, CGI1746, in the active site of Bruton's Tyrosine Kinase (BTK) (in house data; for more details see Di Paolo et al. 2011). This structure was highly relevant because it showed that the binding mode of this competitive inhibitor was quite distinct from irreversible BTK inhibitors, such as ibrutinib, that bind covalently to a cysteine residue (cysteine-481). Computational docking – based on experimentally obtained crystal structures – has proven to be valuable to make more informed drug design decisions, but it is still impossible to predict binding potency with a high degree of accuracy. However, docking is useful to test hypotheses and triage design ideas. Finally, one should always consider that the protein may be flexible and the binding pocket may change depending on the three-dimensional shape of the inhibitor or agonist.

While crystal structures of cytochrome P450 enzymes and transporters (e.g. P-glycoprotein) have been obtained, their use in drug discovery to optimize ADME properties has been limited – to a large extent due to the large active site and promiscuity of these proteins. An elegant exception is a recent study where the authors successfully used the crystal structure of cytochrome P450 2D6 (CYP2D6), a polymorphic enzyme with a relatively small and well-defined active site, to confirm the sites of metabolism of a CK1ε inhibitor and subsequently dial out metabolism by CYP2D6 (Vaz et al. 2018).

Fig. 2.1 (**a**) Crystal structure of CGI1746 in the active site of Bruton's Tyrosine Kinase. (**b**) Molecular structure of CGI1746. (In house data; for more details see Di Paolo et al. 2011)

(a)

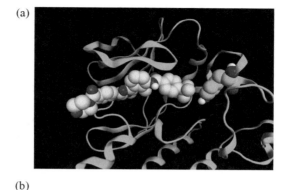

(b)

CGI1746

   Overall, structure-based design is very important and having crystal and co-crystal structures early in drug discovery can greatly advance a project by guiding drug design.

2.1.2   Property-Based Design

Property-based design is based on the observation that most successful drugs have molecular properties within a well-defined and relatively narrow range. Properties that should be considered are: molecular weight, lipophilicity (logP, logD), charge state (pK_a), hydrogen bond donors and acceptors, polar surface area, degree of planarity (number of (aromatic) rings and rotatable bonds, percentage sp^3 carbons), etc. The earliest and most well-known analysis was performed by Chris Lipinski at Pfizer and it resulted in the famous and valuable 'rule of 5' for oral absorption (Table 2.1; Lipinski et al. 1997). Additional rules have been defined since then (Table 2.1).
   Subsequently, it has been shown that not only absorption is influenced by these parameters; distribution, metabolism and excretion, in general, are strongly influenced by the physicochemical properties of a drug. Thereafter, these parameters have been used to influence the design of corporate libraries for high throughput screening and, hence, the starting point for many drug discovery projects.

Table 2.1 Guidelines for estimating drug-like space

Name	Criteria
Lipinski's rule (also known as the rule of 5; Ro5)[11] (Lipinski 2004)	HBD <5 HBA <10 MW <500 Da logP <5
Veber's rule For Oral Drugs[12] (Veber et al. 2002)	Rotatable bonds <10 PSA <140 Å^2
Ghose Filter[13] (Ghose et al. 1999)	MW = 160–480 Da logP between −0.4 and + 5.6 Atom count between 20 and 70 Molar refractivity between 40 and 130
Hughes's rule For higher in vivo safety[14] (Hughes et al. 2008)	logP <3 PSA >75 Å^2
Ritchie's rule For higher developability (lower attrition)[15] (Ritchie and Macdonald 2009)	Number aromatic rings >3

HBA hydrogen bond acceptors (sum of N and O atoms), *HBD* hydrogen bond donors (sum of N–H and O–H bonds), *PSA* polar surface area

Many analyses have been performed looking at the impact of physicochemical parameters on the drug discovery process and numerous correlations have been found. Although some companies hesitate to pursue compounds that violate one or more components of the 'rule of 5' or related rules, the goal of these guidelines should not be to rule out a broad swath of chemical space. After all, several successful drugs violate the 'rule of 5' to some extent; for example, atorvastatin, montelukast, many antiviral agents, prodrugs, and natural products, such as cyclosporine and paclitaxel, all violate one or more of the 'rules'. These guidelines are intended to steer the synthetic chemistry effort towards chemical space that is **more likely** to yield drugs with **superior** ADME properties. Indeed, drugs can be found in 'beyond rule of 5 space', but optimization may take much longer. ADME properties should be considered hand-in-hand with potency data because it is the combination of the two that will ultimately determine the dose. A brief summary of the physicochemical properties of older marketed oral drugs relative to Lipinski's 'rule of 5' is presented in Table 2.2. Other authors have advocated the importance of other physicochemical parameters on ADME: (topological) polar surface area, number of aromatic rings, percentage sp^3 carbons, number of rotatable bonds and higher numbers for all four properties generally result in worse PK properties (Table 2.1).

While most older drugs are generally 'rule of 5' compliant, several authors have shown that the molecular weight and lipophilicity of approved drugs have been gradually increasing (Table 2.2). This has been attributed to the singular focus on high throughput screening and the subsequent push in lead optimization for more and more potent compounds; it has been shown that potency increases with molecular weight and logP in a statistically significant fashion (Gleeson et al. 2011). In the process, compounds may have been optimized to increase lipophilic interactions resulting in mainly entropically-driven (ΔS) gains in potency rather than specific

Table 2.2 Average physicochemical properties of older marketed oral drugs and oral drugs in phase I in comparison with Lipinski's 'rule of 5'

	Phase I oral drugs	Marketed oral drugs	Oral drugs launched pre-1983	Oral drugs launched 1983–2002	Lipinski's 'rule of 5'
MW (Da)	423	337	331	377	≤ 500
clogP	2.6	2.5	2.3	2.5	≤ 5
clogD$_{7.4}$	1.3	1.0			
# of HBDs	2.5	2.1	1.8	1.8	≤ 5
# of HBAs	6.4	4.9	3.0	3.7	≤ 10
NRB	7.8	5.9	5.0	6.4	
Number of rings			2.6	2.9	

Wenlock et al. (2003); Leeson and Davis (2004)
clogP calculated lipophilicity when the compound is neutral
clogD$_{7.4}$ calculated lipophilicity at a pH of 7.4

interactions that drive enthalpically-driven (ΔH) gains in potency. This is what the lipophilic ligand efficiency (LLE)/lipophilic efficiency (LipE) concept attempts to address (Eq. 2.1).

$$LLE = LipE = \ log\big(potency\big) - logD_{7.4} \qquad (2.1)$$

The real goal is to optimize potency without increasing lipophilicity; LLE/LipE values of 7–8 are generally desirable. Another reason for the shift in molecular properties is that many recent drug targets have less well-defined binding pockets that may necessitate larger molecules to attain sufficient potency. The increase in molecular weight and, in particular, lipophilicity has invariably a negative impact on ADME properties. For example, high lipophilicity frequently results in poor solubility, which negatively affects absorption. Also, more lipophilic compounds tend to be more metabolically labile resulting in higher clearance and lower exposure. Indeed, the authors of this book have shown that a higher percentage of compounds with 'rule of 5' violations attrited in development for pharmacokinetic reasons than compounds that are 'rule of 5' compliant (unpublished results). Similarly, an analysis of a database of oral drugs and the ChEMBL database of 'hits' indicated that the mean molecular weights of drugs and 'hits' are 333 and 430 Da, respectively, and the mean logP values are 2.5 and 3.5, respectively (Gleeson et al. 2011). Collectively, these data suggest that poor physicochemical properties and 'rule of 5' violations are **statistically** associated with higher attrition in drug discovery and development and, therefore, physicochemical properties should feature prominently in drug design. Moreover, it has been shown that both high lipophilicity and poor solubility are associated with higher variability in pharmacokinetic studies (Daublain et al. 2017) – mainly driven by variability in absorption. High variability can be quite problematic in clinical development because the exposure may be too low in some patients to achieve efficacy and too high in other patients resulting in toxicity. It is interesting to note that some physicochemical properties influence pharmacokinetic

deutetrabenazine   deucravacitinib

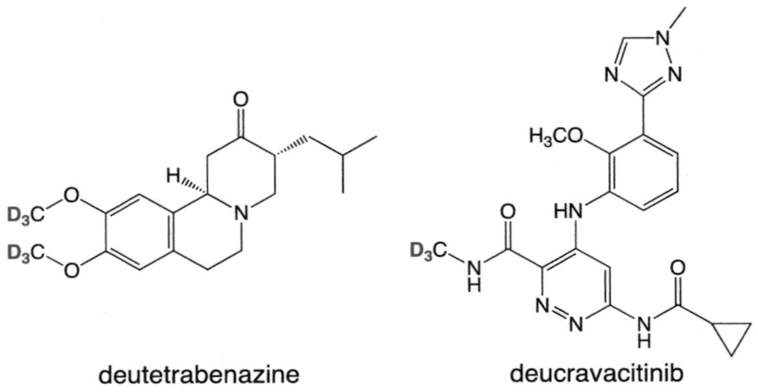

Fig. 2.2 Molecular structures of deuterated compounds deutetrabenazine, a vesicular monoamine transporter 2 inhibitor, and deucravacitinib, a TYK2 inhibitor

properties in opposing ways. For example, increasing the lipophilicity increases the unbound clearance as described above, but it also increases the unbound volume of distribution (Broccatelli et al. 2019). The net result is actually a small increase in half-life with increasing lipophilicity. Of course, increasing the lipophilicity could also come at the expense of solubility and decreased absorption. The winning strategy is usually identifying and fixing a specific site of metabolism without a concomitant change in lipophilicity and adversely affecting other pharmacokinetic parameters. One such attempt involves the replacement of hydrogen atoms with deuterium atoms to improve metabolic stability; C-D bonds are slightly stronger than C-H bonds (see Sect. 2.4.4). Deutetrabenazine, a vesicular monoamine transporter 2 inhibitor, has been approved and deucravacitinib, a TYK2 inhibitor, is in phase 3 clinical trials (Fig. 2.2). Often, various physicochemical properties have an inter-related impact on pharmacokinetic properties and the drug discovery process usually involves iterative design and synthesis of hundreds to thousands of compounds before identifying the one molecule that has the right **balance** of properties and this process usually involves a level of **compromise**.

Other important considerations are the molecular target in question, its location and the route of administration. For example, if a project is intended to disrupt complex protein-protein interaction, it is particularly unlikely to stay within the 'rule of 5'. A nice example is venetoclax, a selective Bcl2 inhibitor for the treatment of chronic lymphocytic leukemia and small lymphocytic lymphoma (Fig. 2.3). Its molecular properties are rather extreme: the logP is 8.9, the MW is 868 Da and the topological polar surface area (TPSA) is 172 $Å^2$. Not surprisingly, the solubility is essentially zero in buffer, but fortunately much higher in lipid-based solvents (solubility in soybean oil is 2.2 mg/mL). Considering the nature of the target, it was impossible to identify a drug that would comply with the 'rule of 5'. Inevitably, optimization of the ADME properties was a central component of the screening cascade and time-consuming; considering the complex pharmacokinetics, *in vitro* models were not particularly predictive and, therefore, a large number of *in vivo* PK studies were performed and this involved extensive formulation optimization. Somewhat surprisingly, the oral bioavailability of venetoclax was close to 40% in fed

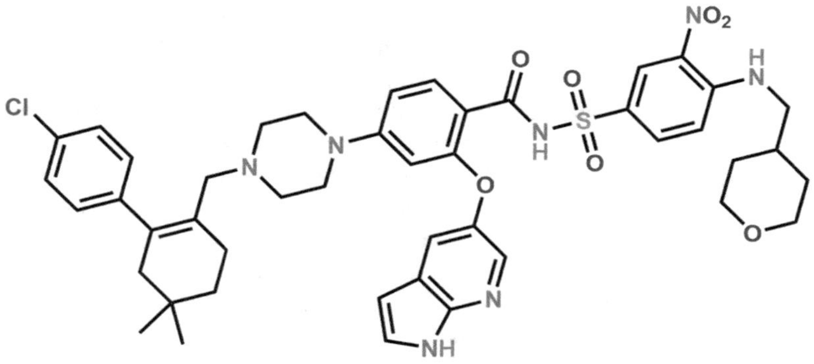

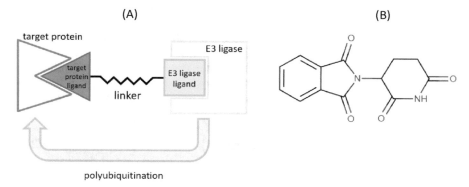

Fig. 2.3 Molecular structure of venetoclax, a selective Bcl2 inhibitor

(A)   (B)

Fig. 2.4 (**a**) Depiction of the structure of a bifunctional protein degrader and (**b**) the molecular structure of the cereblon ligand thalidomide

dogs (Choo et al. 2014) and the oral exposure in humans was remarkably good (Salem et al. 2016). Subsequently, it was shown by Choo et al. 2014 that about half of the absorption in dogs (and presumably in humans) is driven by lymphatic absorption, which in turn is fueled by the extreme lipophilicity of venetoclax. In general, candidates for lymphatic absorption are characterized by high lipophilicity (log P >5) and lipid solubility (≥50 mg/mL). Not surprisingly, the exposure of venetoclax increases with a high fat meal because it improves the solubility (Salem et al. 2016). While the human dose of venetoclax is reasonable, 400 mg, the large amount of excipients required to improve solubilization inevitably results in a higher pill burden (4 pills a day). The pill burden should be considered in drug development because a high pill burden is usually correlated with reduced compliance and, hence, efficacy.

Bifunctional protein (chimeric) degraders are another class of compounds that have garnered a lot of attention recently, but are not 'rule of 5'compliant (see Sect. 2.4.6). These degraders are comprised of three parts as shown in Fig. 2.4a: a ligand of the target of interest, a linker and, for example, an E3 ligase ligand (VHL or cereblon). The concept is that the bifunctional degrader will bring the target and the ligase in close proximity, which will result in ubiquitination of the target of interest and, subsequently, degradation of the target in the proteasome. If the re-synthesis rate of the target is sufficiently long (e.g. >24 h), degradation of the target is an attractive approach to reduce or eliminate its role in disease. Of course, the inevitable molecular complexity will result in high molecular weight molecules (>800 Da), which makes absorption and oral bioavailability challenging. To some extent, this has been overcome by reducing the size and number of hydrogen bond donors and acceptors in the E3 ligase ligand. Indeed, cereblon ligands, such as thalidomide analogs (see Fig. 2.4b), are generally more likely to result in an orally bioavailable bifunctional degrader. More details about the optimization process required for bifunctional protein degraders are provided in Edmondson et al. 2019 and Cantrill et al. 2020.

These are just some of the examples illustrating that drugs can be found in 'beyond rule of 5 space' and that some targets make exploration of this chemical space inevitable. Indeed, the trend of increasing molecular complexity observed from pre-1983 to 1983–2002 (Table 2.2) has increased further in most recent years – as illustrated in Table 2.3. Between 2013 and 2017 more than half of the approved drugs had a molecular weight of more than 500 Da, clearly indicating that a molecular weight cut off of 500 Da may not be critical. DeGoey et al. 2018 came to the same conclusion. They reviewed the relation between rat oral bioavailability and various physicochemical parameters and proposed a new 'rule' for oral bioavailability (or lack thereof) to evaluate 'beyond rule of 5' compounds that is less rigid than Lipinski's 'rule of five' – see Eq. 2.2.

$$AB\text{-}MPS = Abs(cLogD - 3) + NAR + NRB \qquad (2.2)$$

AB-MPS = Abbvie multiparametric score
Abs = absolute value
cLogD = calculated lipophilicity
NAR = number of aromatic rings
NRB = number of rotatable bonds

Table 2.3 Mean physicochemical properties of oral drugs approved by the FDA from 1998 to 2007 and 2008 to 2017 in comparison with Lipinski's 'rule of 5'

	Drugs approved from 1998 to 2007	Drugs approved from 2008 to 2017	Lipinski's 'rule of 5'
MW (Da)	360	437	≤500
clogP	2.4	2.9	≤5
TPSA (Å)	82	94	
# of HBDs	1.8	2.1	≤5
# of HBAs	6.0	6.8	≤10
NRB	5.9	7.0	
# of aromatic rings	1.7	2.2	

Shultz (2019)
clogP calculated lipophilicity when the compound is neutral

An AB-MPS score of ≤14 predicts a higher probability of oral absorption and molecular weight does not appear in the AB-MPS score because it is deemed more forgiving than originally thought. It is noteworthy that almost all the bifunctional protein degraders highlighted in Edmondson et al. 2019 had AB-MPS scores in excess of 20 indicating that oral bioavailability remains challenging for these compounds. Finally, while there may be more room for success beyond the 'rule of 5' than originally anticipated, the number of approved oral drugs that violate two or more of the rules is small; only 17% of the oral drugs approved between 2010 and 2019 violated two or more of the rules (Brown and Wobst 2021). In conclusion, for some targets it is impossible to stay within the 'rule of 5', but this usually results in far more ADME and formulation optimization, which can be quite time consuming. Exquisite potency can be a compensating factor. Indeed, each target may have a unique physicochemical sweet spot that needs to be incorporated in design of new leads. Excellent overviews with many examples of 'beyond rule of 5' drugs are Doak et al. 2014 and DeGoey et al. 2018.

Many natural products that are orally absorbed are not 'rule of 5' compliant. An example is cyclosporine A, an immunosuppressant for the treatment of rheumatoid arthritis, psoriasis and Crohn's disease. The physiochemical properties of cyclosporine would suggest poor absorption.

However, the oral bioavailability in humans is about 30%. The latter is due to its chameleonic character where cyclosporine forms hydrogen bond interactions with water in solution and it forms intramolecular hydrogen bonds when it permeates across a membrane. A detailed nuclear magnetic resonance (NMR) and gas phase computational analysis has shown that cyclosporine forms 4 internal hydrogen bonds, which reduces the number of hydrogen bond donors from 5 to 1 (Alex et al. 2011). Cyclosporine is also a substrate of various transporters.

Cyclosporine A
MW = 1202 Da
clogP = 4.0
TPSA = 279 Å^2
HBD = 5
HBA = 12

Table 2.4 Important factors based on Biopharmaceutics Drug Disposition Classification System (BDDCS) that captures predominant mechanisms of clearance from metabolism to transport

	High solubility	Low solubility
High permeability	1: Metabolism	2: Metabolism
		Efflux transporter
	Elimination by metabolism	
Low permeability	3: Renal/biliary	4: Renal/biliary
	Absorptive transport effect	Absorptive/efflux transport
	Elimination of unchanged drug	

Wu and Benet (2005)

Physicochemical parameters can also be used to bin compounds and facilitate identification of processes involved in drug disposition. Prof. Leslie Benet proposed the Biopharmaceutics Drug Disposition Classification System (BDDCS; Wu and Benet 2005), which is derived from the Biopharmaceutics Classification System (BCS). This classification system can be used to identify the rate-determining step in drug elimination – metabolism vs efflux or uptake transporters (Table 2.4). This concept describes compounds in BDDCS class 1 and 2 (highly permeable) as mainly metabolized with class 1 drugs having minimal transporter involvement and efflux drug transport may occur for class 2 drugs. For Class 3 and 4 drugs (poorly permeable), metabolism is minimal and drug transporters are major contributors. Conceptually, high permeability is correlaterd with metabolic clearance pathways in the liver. In addition, there are also proposals to replace solubility with PSA or other parameters (Chankhamjon et al. 2019; Di et al. 2013). With lower permeability, drug transport is more likely involved with drug distribution and ultimately elimination. Note that BDDCS does not differentiate metabolic pathways.

The Biopharmaceutics Classification System (BCS)
- HIGHLY SOLUBLE: the highest dose is soluble in equal or less than 250 ml water over a pH of 1 to 7.5.
- HIGHLY PERMEABLE: absorption in humans is >90%
- RAPIDLY DISSOLVING when greater than 85% of the drug dissolves within 30 min

http://www.fda.gov/cder/OPS/BCS_guidance.htm

Scientists at Pfizer proposed a more sophisticated classification system: the Extended Clearance Classification System (ECCS; Varma et al. 2015) that looks at the impact of permeability and charge state on drug disposition (Fig. 2.5). The nature of the target to be inhibited or agonized will usually lock in the chemical space for a particular project. However, it is generally preferred if metabolism is the

Class	major route of clearance	permeability	ionization	MW
1A	metabolism	high	acid, zwitterion	≤400
1B	hepatic uptake-transport	high	acid, zwitterion	>400
2	metabolism	high	base, neutral	wide range
3A	renal	low	acid, zwitterion	≤400
3B	hepatic uptake-transport or renal	low	acid, zwitterion	>400
4	renal	low	base, neutral	wide range

Fig. 2.5 Extended clearance classification system (ECCS) that captures predominant mechanisms of clearance from metabolism to transport. Permeability cut off 5×10^{-6} cm/s in MDCK. (Varma et al. 2015)

rate determining step and the main route of drug elimination because *in vitro – in vivo* correlation (IVIVC) is well established for metabolism using microsomes/S9/hepatocytes and IVIVC of transporter substrates is prone to underestimation of human clearance.

Further refinement of the ECCS classification system (El-Kattan and Varma 2018):

- Classes 1B and 3B drugs are likely prone to OATP-mediated hepatic uptake.
- Classes 3A, 4 and certain class 3B drugs are predominantly cleared renally and OAT1, OAT3, OCT2 and MATEs could contribute to their active renal secretion.
- Intestinal efflux and uptake transporters largely influence the oral pharmacokinetics of class 3A, 3B and 4 drugs.

It is very important to keep in mind that these classification systems, as well as other correlations, are based on statistical significance, but they are far from perfect and exceptions exist. Nevertheless, they can help guide the focus of a drug discovery effort and help identify assays to prioritize in the screening cascade during lead optimization.

CNS Drugs

For central nervous system (CNS) drugs that need to cross the blood-brain barrier, the criteria are and remain stricter than for non-CNS drugs: a molecular weight below 400 Da, number of hydrogen bond donors below 3, and a topological polar surface area below <90 Å² are desirable. See Table 2.5 for more details about the

Table 2.5 Average physicochemical properties of oral CNS drugs in phase I and marketed drugs in comparison with Lipinski's and Pajouhseh's rules for CNS compounds

	Oral CNS drugs launched 1983–2002	Oral CNS drugs launched 1983–2002	Lipinski's rule for CNS compounds	Pajouhseh's rule for CNS compounds
MW (Da)	310	377	≤400	<450
clogP	2.5	2.5	≤5	<5
clogD$_{7.4}$				
# of *HBDs*	1.5	1.8	≤3	<3
# of *HBAs*	2.1	3.7	≤7	<7
# of *RBs*	4.7	6.4		<8
# of aromatic rings	2.9	2.9		
PSA (Å^2)				60–90
% PSA	16	21		
pK$_a$				7.5–10.5

Leeson and Davis (2004); Pajouhesh and Lenz (2005)

physicochemical properties for oral CNS drugs. Beyond those limits, crossing the blood-brain barrier is harder and/or the compounds are more likely to be substrates of efflux transporters like P-glycoprotein (P-gp) and breast cancer resistance protein (BCRP). Indeed, P-gp efflux out of the brain increases dramatically with an increasing number of hydrogen bond donors, because it is these hydrogen bond donors that interact with hydrogen bond acceptors in P-gp.

> Most of the inhaled compounds used for the treatment of asthma are 'rule of 5' compliant and the structures of a few drugs are provided below. Many of them have low solubility, which results in slow release and therefore, a long-acting effect. In contrast, the short acting bronchodilator, ipratropium, is charged and has high solubility. Once absorbed in the lung and released in the systemic circulation, a high rate of metabolism is preferred to avoid any systemic side effects. Since a significant fraction of an inhaled drug reaches the stomach and the intestine, most inhaled drugs are designed to have a high rate of first pass metabolism.
>
> Structures of fluticasone and budesonide, both inhaled corticosteroid, and salmeterol, a long-acting beta agonist and ipratropium, a short acting bronchodilator:

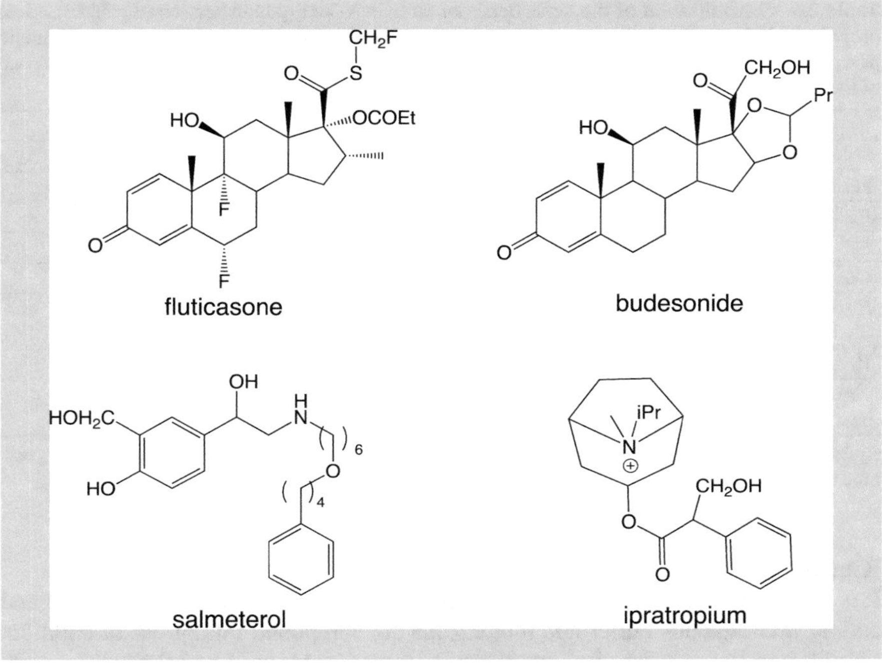

In summary, the dependence of various ADME properties on physicochemical parameters is described in Table 2.6 and it can be used as a guide in design of compounds with superior ADME properties. While drugs can be found in 'beyond rule of 5' chemical space, the following remains valuable advice: *"Where there is a choice in a therapeutic area between a lipophilic agent that violates the rules and one with a better balance of properties, senior management would still be best advised to back the latter. Imperfect agents might simply validate a target and encourage competitors to enter with a drug having the improved properties."* (Teague 2011).

2.2 Solubility

Solubility is particularly important in drug discovery and depends on parameters such as lipophilicity and pK_a. While solubility is relatively easy to determine, it also depends highly on both the form of the material and the assay conditions. There are two types of solubility measurements: kinetic and thermodynamic solubility.

Table 2.6 Generalization of the dependence of various ADME parameters on physicochemical properties. The arrows indicate an increase, no change or decrease of the pharmacokinetic parameter in one of the rows as a function of an increase in the physiochemical parameter in one of the columns

	logD	MW	PSA	HBA + HBD
Solubility	↓	↓	↑	↑
Permeability	↑	↓	↓	↓
F_a	↑	↓	↓	↓
F_h	↓	=	↑	↑
CL	↑		↓	↓
F	Gaussian (↑ then ↓)	↓	Gaussian (↑ then ↓)	↓
V_d	↑		↓	↓
Plasma protein binding	↑			

F_a fraction absorbed, F_h fraction absorbed by the liver, CL clearance, F oral bioavailability, V_d volume of distribution

Kinetic Solubility

It is obtained by dissolving the compound in an organic solvent (e.g. DMSO) and adding it to aqueous buffer and looking for the compound falling out of solution. Equilibrium is not reached between the dissolved compound and the solid, which may also not be the most stable polymorph. Kinetic solubility measurements are easy to perform and useful to assess solubility issues encountered in routine *in vitro* potency and ADME assays. However, kinetic solubility measurements are of limited relevance to the situation encountered *in vivo*.

Thermodynamic Solubility

It is obtained by adding the aqueous buffer directly to solid crystalline material and waiting for an extended period of time for equilibrium between the dissolved and solid material. Although thermodynamic solubility is more relevant, it consumes more material and the measurement is time consuming. Solubility also depends on the medium; thermodynamic solubility is usually measured in buffer, fasted state simulated intestinal fluid (FaSSIF; pH ≈ 6.5) and fed state simulated intestinal fluid (FeSSIF; pH ≈ 5). For example, felodipine is 100-fold more soluble in FeSSIF than in water and is not pH dependent in water. Finally, solubility depends on the pH of the medium. Basic compounds are ionized at lower pH and, therefore, more soluble in the stomach, but the solubility may be much lower at higher pH in the intestine and the compound may crash out. For acids, the opposite occurs and the solubility is low in the stomach, but higher in the intestine. Not only is the extent of solubility important, the rate should be taken into consideration as well. The dissolution rate can be assessed in thermodynamic solubility experiments.

The material obtained in the first synthesis of a compound is frequently poorly characterized and, especially for more lipophilic compounds, amorphous. An amorphous compound may have decent solubility in the kinetic solubility assay, but it could change dramatically once converted to a crystalline form and determined in a thermodynamic solubility assay. Salt form and polymorph screens are performed later in drug discovery and also in development. An infamous example is ritonavir, an antiretroviral compound for the treatment of HIV. Ritonavir was approved in 1996 and this involved what is now called form I. However, another, more stable form, form II, was discovered in 1998 and this form was less soluble resulting in lower oral bioavailability and, hence, exposure. Moreover, a trace amount of form II accelerated conversion of form I into form II. In the end, the capsules were withdrawn and patients had to switch to the suspension. After a large amount of formulation work, Abbvie switched to a refrigerated gelcap. Finally, it may be possible to improve the solubility and/or dissolution rate by changing the salt form, reducing the particle size or modifying the formulation. Adding excipients, such as in amorphous spray dried dispersions, can improve the oral bioavailability, but it also increases the pill burden. Amorphous spray dried dispersion is usually only a practical solution up to a dose of 250 mg of the active ingredient.

2.3 Multi-Parameter Optimization (MPO)

Ultimately, drug discovery is an exercise in multi-parameter optimization (MPO). In the previous section, the tradeoffs between potency and ADME properties were discussed. In reality, the picture is far more complex and off-target activity as well as *in vitro* and *in vivo* toxicity endpoints need to be incorporated as well. To date, this optimization process has been guided by experienced 'drug hunters', usually medicinal chemists, with input from many functional leads in departments such as *in vitro* and *in vivo* pharmacology, drug metabolism & pharmacokinetics, preclinical toxicology, etc. Once a project is close to delivering a development candidate, sensitivity analyses using physiologically-based pharmacokinetic modeling and pharmacokinetic/pharmacodynamic modeling can be performed to identify those parameters that influence the human dose most and, hence, the viability of a particular lead (see Chap. 4). However, simpler MPO tools are needed early on in drug discovery. The goal should not be a perfect prediction; instead, these MPO tools should be used for prioritization of leads in the optimization process.

Humans, even experienced 'drug hunters', can at most consider three parameters reliably in a parallel optimization process. With advances in computational tools, this has become much easier and computational models are quite adept at sifting through thousands, if not millions, of data points and identifying compounds with a greater **likelihood** of succeeding. That said, the scoring functions that are the

Case 2.1: Isosteres to Improve Solubility

Tioconazole has poor solubility and it is used for topical applications. Adding more polarity to improve solubility allowed for the discovery of **fluconazole** for systemic administration and the treatment of fungal infections. (Richardson et al. 1990)

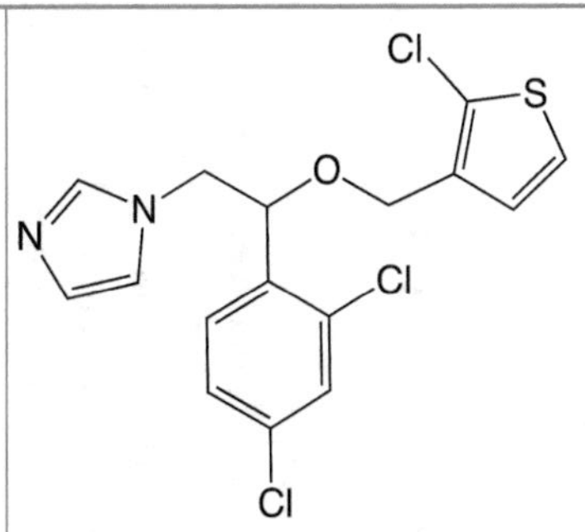

tioconazole

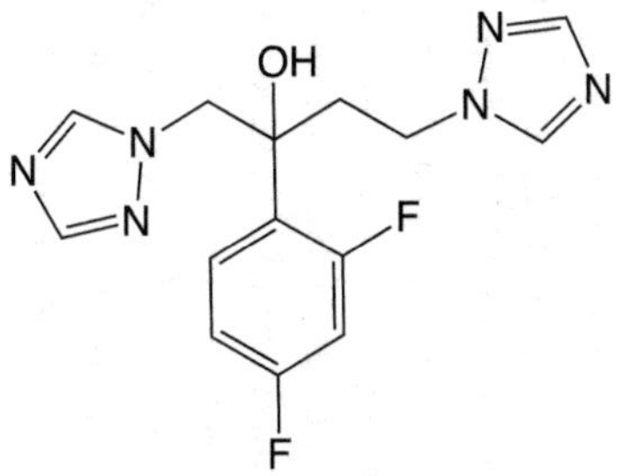

fluconazole

foundation of any MPO tool still require input from experts. Most recently, the use of deep neural networks has shown to be useful for the identification of new drug candidates. While there is a lot of hype about artificial intelligence (AI), the methodology is useful for identifying candidates for established targets with a lot of data in the public domain. AI is less successful in novel chemical space and/or for new targets. The one area where AI has shown its value is for ADME optimization where companies have large quantities of data generated under identical conditions (Bhhatarai et al. 2019). See Sect. 3.2 for more details.

An attractive way for MPO that incorporates both potency and the ADME perspective is predicting the human efficacious dose. It is important to distinguish the detailed human PK and dose predictions that are done just before candidate nominations, and the predictions that can be done – with various assumptions – much earlier in the drug discovery process to prioritize compounds. For example, Eq. 2.3 provides a very simple and useful model to predict the human dose and it incorporates parameters that are commonly available in drug discovery:

$$\text{Dose} = C_{avg,ss} \times CL \times \tau / F \tag{2.3}$$

$C_{avg,ss}$: average steady state concentration and defined here by the *in vitro* potency, e.g. IC_{50}, divided by the free fraction in plasma

CL: predicted hvuman clearance – usually derived from human liver microsomes or hepatocytes or other scaling methods

τ: dosing interval (usually 12 or 24 h)

F: back-calculated bioavailability assuming that the clearance is solely hepatic (1 – CL/Q) or based on preclinical bioavailability data

In this model, the average steady state concentration, $C_{avg,ss}$, is the determinant of the dose. This is usually a good starting point, but considerable debate remains whether IC_{50}/EC_{50}, IC_{70}/EC_{70} or IC_{90}/EC_{90} values should be used; of course, the choice depends heavily on the nature of the target. Eq. 2.4 describes a more complex scenario and needs more input parameters (Page 2016).

$$\text{Dose} = \left(\frac{MEC_{ss} \times AR \times \left(k_a - k_{elim} \right) \times V_d}{k_a \times \left(e^{-k_{elim} \times \tau} - e^{k_a \times \tau} \right)} \right) \Big/ F \tag{2.4}$$

MEC_{ss}: minimum effective concentration (i.e., potency corrected for protein binding) at steady state

AR: accumulation ratio = $1 - e^{-k_{elim} \times \tau}$

k_a: absorption rate

k_{elim}: elimination rate

V_d: volume of distribution

τ: dosing interval (usually 12 or 24 h)

F: bioavailability

Models can be derived using the following drivers of efficacy: AUC, $C_{max,ss}$, $C_{avg,ss}$, $C_{min,ss}$, or any other time over threshold. The $C_{min,ss}$ – the concentration at 24 h for QD dosing and the concentration at 12 h for BID dosing – approach is the most conservative because it requires continuous coverage of the *in vitro* potency, be it IC_{50}/EC_{50}, IC_{70}/EC_{70} or IC_{90}/EC_{90}. However, it requires prediction of the whole pharmacokinetic curve and, in particular, the concentration at trough, which is usually more variable and fraught with error. More details about various simple dose predictions methods are presented in Maurer et al. 2020. Again, it is important to emphasize that these models are not meant to be an accurate dose prediction. It is merely meant to provide an indication about the order of magnitude and a means to help **prioritize** compounds for further study. Once a lead has been identified, more detailed *in vitro* and *in vivo* studies can be performed and the corresponding data can be incorporated in a physiologically-based pharmacokinetic model to predict the human pharmacokinetics and then a pharmacokinetic/pharmacodynamic model to predict the human dose.

The extent of target coverage required for efficacy in humans remains a popular and critical topic of debate. Indeed, if a larger degree of target coverage is required, the dose will go up significantly. It is common to attempt to relate the clinically efficacious exposure to the potency measured in *in vitro* assays. (As described elsewhere in this book, it is important to convert any *in vitro* potency value to a relevant *in vivo* efficacious exposure by correcting it for protein binding in both the *in vitro* incubation medium and *in vivo* plasma.) Both Smith and Rowland 2019 and Jansson-Löfmark et al. 2020 have shown that on average equating the average unbound steady state concentration in humans with either IC_{50}, EC_{50} or K_i seems the most appropriate descriptor of the driver of efficacy. There is considerable uncertainty and variability in this assessment and the situation is very much dependent on the specifics of each molecular target and the *in vitro* assay conditions. For example, IC_{50}/EC_{50} coverage appears sufficient for efficacy with kinase inhibitors, whereas much more target coverage, $\geq IC_{90}/EC_{90}$, is required for anti-infectives (mostly to prevent resistance) and agonists may require less than IC_{50}/EC_{50}.

2.4 Drug Properties and Therapeutic Targets

Here we highlight some large drug classes and their therapeutic targets. In general, the medicine (drug intervention) is geared towards reversing or at least minimizing the impact of the disease state. For this reason, many types of molecules (modalities) can be deployed and here we capture several types (Fig. 2.6).

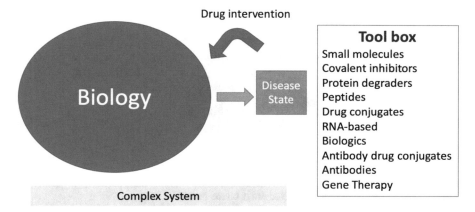

Fig. 2.6 Drug intervention allows reversing or minimizing disease state and for this purpose multitude of molecules (modalities) are deployed

2.4.1 G Protein-Coupled Receptor (GPCR)-Targeted Drugs

G protein-coupled receptors (GPCRs) comprise the largest family of membrane receptors that are targeted by FDA approved drugs. More than 130 approved drugs are targeting GPCRs (Fig. 2.7; Sriram and Insel 2018).

Modes of binding: Agonists, antagonists, or allosteric modulators.

Targets: GPCRs mediate cellular responses to most hormones, metabolites, cytokines and neurotransmitters. They modulate several signaling processes involved in behavior, blood pressure regulation, cognition, immune response, mood, smell and taste (Thomsen et al. 2005).

Structure: Seven transmembrane domain receptors linked by three extracellular (ECL) and three intracellular (ICL) loops (Ciancetta et al. 2015). GPCRs are detectable from outside the cell and activated by cell-surface binding leading to cellular responses.

Classes: GPCRs are categorized into six classes based on sequence and function. Class A = rhodopsin-like receptors, Class B = secretin family, Class C = metabotropic glutamate receptors, Class D = fungal mating pheromone receptors, Class E = cAMP receptors, and Class F = frizzled (FZD) and smoothened (SMO) receptors.

Professor Alfred Goodman Gilman won the Nobel prize in physiology or medicine in 1994 in recognition of the discovery of G-proteins, which allow chemical signals to be transmitted to the interior of cells.

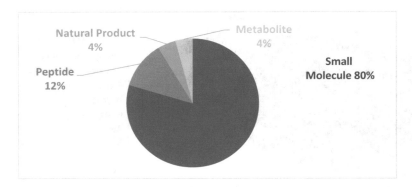

Fig. 2.7 Classification of GPCR-targeted drugs on the market

dacomitinib* (2018)	erdafitinib (2018)	cobimetinib (2015)
lenvatinib (2015)	afatinib* (2013)	ibrutinib* (2013)

Fig. 2.8 Examples of FDA approved kinase inhibitors from 2013 to 2018. (*covalent modifiers)

2.4.2 Kinase Inhibitors

Kinase inhibitors represent an important therapeutic class with more than 30 registered drugs (Fig. 2.8). Kinases are enzymes that conjugates a phosphate (PO_4) group to a protein, and hence modulate its function. The donor of phosphate is the high energy ATP and therefore kinases have an ATP binding site. The amino acids modified in the phosphorolation process are commonly to serine, threonine, or tyrosine on the protein (in addition there is histidine). Phosphorylation regulates many biological processes, and protein kinase inhibitors can be used to treat diseases due to hyperactive protein kinases (including mutant or overexpressed kinases in cancer) or to modulate cell functions to overcome other disease drivers. Despite the hundreds of kinase proteins that exist in humans, most of them have an active site that is similar in structure and function. The first marketed drug in this class was imatinib, which was approved by the FDA in 2001. The physicochemical properties that define drug-like kinase inhibitors are shown in Table 2.7. Most kinase inhibitor have been developed for cancer indications, but the usage of kinases is expanding to include immunology (e.g., tofacitinib).

Table 2.7 Summary of average properties of kinase inhibitors

Properties	Limits	% Kinases within this limit
MW (Da)	<500	70
LogP	1–5	80
	>5	20
HBD	≤3	97
HBA	≤8	85
Rotatable bonds	≤10	100
PSA (Å²)	≤140	100
	≤100	73
pKa	≤8	64
	8–9	29
	>9	7
BCS	I	10
	II	52
	III	7
	IV	27
Substrate of transport	One or more Pgp and BCRP efflux transporters	80
Bioavailability (%)	>20% across all reported species	76
V_{ss} (L/kg)	0.28 to 43.6 Basic inhibitors (~33%; pKa >9) V_{ss} >10 L/kg.	Majority with limited CNS penetration

O'Brien and Moghaddam (2017)

BCS Biopharmaceutical Classification System, *CNS* central nervous system, *HBA* hydrogen bond acceptors, *HBD* hydrogen bond donors, *PSA* polar surface area, *Vss* volume of distribution at steady state

Case 2.2: Discovery of Macrocycle lorlatinib from Crizotinib Using Structure-Based Drug Design

Crizotinib is a first generation small molecule Anaplastic lymphoma kinase (ALK) inhibitor (ATP competitive). It was further optimized using a structure-based drug design approach that resulted in the discovery of the macrocycle product, lorlatinib. Lorlatinib has improved p-gp efflux and metabolic stability compared to crizotinib and overcomes ALK mutant resistance (Johnson et al. 2014; Akamine et al. 2018).

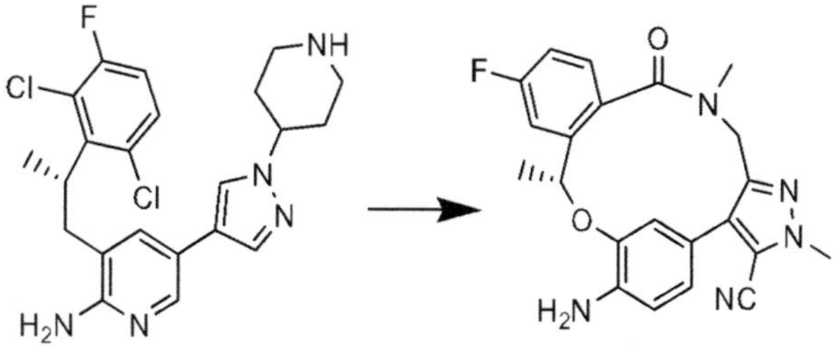

Crizotinib   Loratinib

2.4.3 Covalent Inhibitors

Covalent inhibitors (CI; also known as covalent modifiers) are drugs that bear a reactive nucleophilic functionality (a warhead) designed to bind covalently to a specific protein target (Fig. 2.9; Baillie 2016; Gehringer and Laufer 2018). CIs can have superior efficacy and improved therapeutic index compared to non-CIs due to prolonged target residence time and occupancy without the need for sustained drug exposures in systemic circulation. Note that CIs are most effective if the natural resynthesis rate of the target is 24 h or more; if resynthesis is rapid (e.g., minutes), CIs and reversible inhibitors will behave the same from an efficacy point of view. The properties of marketed CIs and their structures can be seen in Table 2.8 and Fig. 2.10, respectively.

Types of Reactions

Reversible covalent inhibitors: These inhibitors possess electrophilic moieties with low reactivity that bind to their targets and produce labile cross-linked products that subsequently dissociate from the targets with a rate that is faster than the turnover rate of the protein target.

Irreversible covalent inhibitors: These inhibitors form adducts to their protein targets that either do not dissociate from the protein during its lifetime or dissociate from it with a rate that is significantly slower than the resynthesis rate of the target.

Common target nucleophilic side-chains: cysteine, serine and lysine.

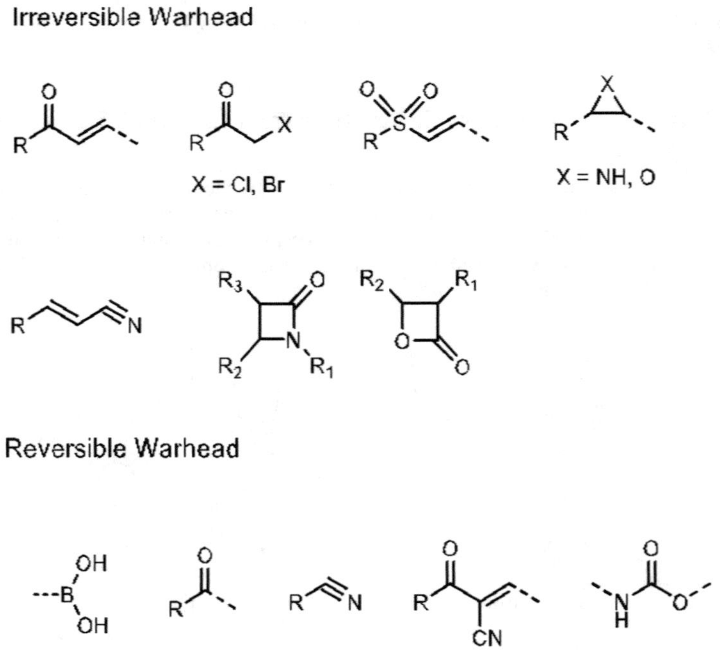

Irreversible Warhead

X = Cl, Br   X = NH, O

Reversible Warhead

Fig. 2.9 Select examples of electrophilic warheads used in covalent inhibitors. (Lagoutte et al. 2017)

Table 2.8 Properties of marketed covalent inhibitors approved by the FDA and/or EMA from 2007–2017

Name (approval year)	T.A.	Target site	Target $t_{1/2}$ (hr)	Dose (mg/day)	CL (mL/min/kg)	V_{ss} (L/ kg)	$t_{1/2}$ (hr)	F/F$_a$ (%)
Vigabatrin **1** (2009)	CNS	Lys-PLP	72	3000	1.0–1.6[a]	1.1[b]	7.5	>60/100
Carfilzomib[c] **2** (2012)	ONC	Thr	30	27 mg/m^2	36–63	0.4	<1.0	NA
Afatinib **3** (2013)	ONC	Cys	16–24	40	13–25[a]	44[b]	37	NA
Ibrutinib **4** (2013)	ONC	Cys	16–24	420	15–18	10	4–6	<5/100
Osimertinib **5** (2015)	ONC	Cys	16–24	80	3.4[a]	14[b]	48	NA/>80
Neratinib **6** (2017)	ONC	Cys	16–24	240	49–63[a]	92[b]	7–17	NA
Acalabrutinib **7** (2017)	ONC	Cys	16–24	200	9	0.5	0.9	25/NA
Avibactam[c] **8** (2015)	ID	Ser	n.a.	1500	2.7–2.9	0.3	2.5	NA
Boceprevir **9** (2011)	ID	Ser	>24	2400	36[a]	11[b]	3.4	NA
Telaprevir **10** (2011)	ID	Ser	>24	2250	7.3[a]	3.6[b]	9–10	NA/>50
Saxagliptin **11** (2009)	MD	Ser	>24	2.5 or 5	7.1	1.7	2.5	>75/>75
Vildagliptin **12** (2007)	MD	Ser	>24	100	9.8	1.0	2–3	85/NA

Excluding prodrugs; Zang et al. (2018)

CL clearance, *CNS* central nervous system, *Cys* cysteine, *ID* infectious diseases, *F* oral bioavailability, *F$_a$* fraction absorbed, *Lys-PLP* lysine-pyridoxal 5'-phosphate cofactor, *MD* metabolic diseases, *ONC* oncology, *Ser* serine, $t_{1/2}$ half-life, *T.A.* therapeutic area, *Thr* threonine, *Vss* volume of distribution at steady state

[a]The CL/F value is reported; [b]The V_{ss}/F value is reported; [c]intravenous route; NA: not available

Stability in whole blood, in addition to liver microsome and hepatocyte stability, is informative for assessing drug reactivity in a physiological relevant environment. The major clearance (CL) mechanisms of covalent inhibitors include both metabolism and renal excretion. Extrahepatic clearance can be a major component of the total clearance. Therefore, relying on only *in vitro* hepatocyte systems could underestimate the overall clearance and overestimate the contribution of CYP metabolism to the overall clearance *in vivo*, potentially resulting in misleading human PK and dose projections.

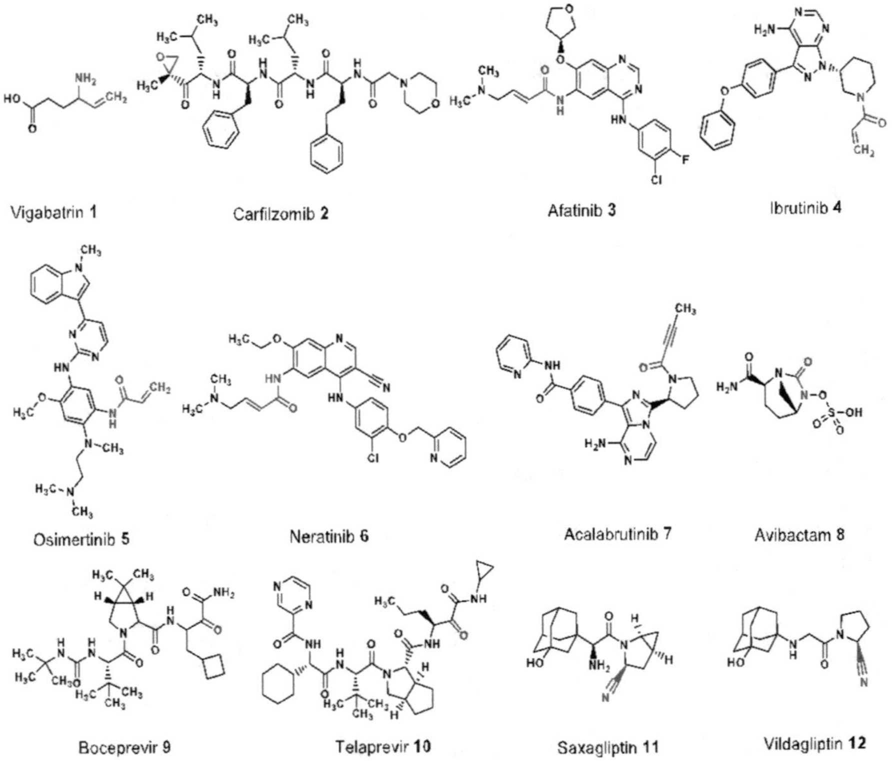

Fig. 2.10 Chemical structures of marketed covalent inhibitors (CIs). Red designates the electrophilic moieties in these CIs

2.4.4   Deuterated Drugs

Drug deuteration replaces a C-H bond with the stronger C-D bond, thus altering the compound's pharmacokinetic properties. Among other benefits, this strategy slows the rate of oxidation that would otherwise proceed via C-H bond cleavage (Johnson et al. 2020).[23] Hence, the replacement of a hydrogen atom with a deuterium atom improves metabolic stability, resulting in reduced drug clearance (Table 2.9). The advantage of drug deuteration is that it avoids major scaffold changes, which may drastically alter the potency and physicochemical and ADME properties of a compound. For that reason, deuterated drugs have become more popular lately.

The Drug Deuteration Process Each deuterated drug candidate should be run through the appropriate *in vitro* metabolism assays prior to dosing *in vivo*. Four key elements should be considered before proceeding with deuteration:

Table 2.9 Challenges solved by deuterium incorporation

ADME challenges	Drug reactions
Lowering CL	Ivacaftor (11 h) ➔ VX-561 (15 h) (Harbeson et al. 2017)
	Ruxolitinib ➔ CTP-534[a]
	Levodopa ➔ SD-1077 (Schneider et al. 2018)
	M9831 (novel) (Harnor et al. 2017)
Improved bioavailability	Dextromethorphan ➔ AVP-786 (Nguyen et al. 2017)
Mitigating a reactive metabolite	Paroxetine ➔ CTP-347 (Uttamsingh et al. 2015)
	Nevirapine ➔ 12-D3-Nevirapine (Heck et al. 2020; Sharma et al. 2013)
	Tamoxifen ➔ D5-Tamoxifen (Phillips et al. 1994)
Slowing chiral inversion	Pioglitazone ➔ DRX-065[b]
Decrease metabolite exposure	JNJ38877605 ➔ D-JNJ38877605 (Zang et al. 2018)

[a]AdisInsight Drugs. (2016) Springer. https://adisinsight.springer.com/drugs/800045309
[b] captured in this poster DeuteRx

1. Target drug metabolizing enzymes: cytochrome P450, aldehyde oxidase and monoamine oxidase
2. Metabolic reaction mechanism: Hydrogen atom abstraction (HAT) needs to be the rate limiting step as determined by the kinetic isotope effect (KIE), which is defined as the change in reaction rate due to isotopic substitution (Fig. 2.11). The compound should undergo no more than two primary metabolic pathways, and these pathways should be mediated by known enzymes. The metabolic reaction has to be compatible with an expected KIE of at least 5 or greater. Non-metabolic clearance pathways, such as renal elimination, should be minor.
3. In vitro stability and contribution to metabolism: The *in vitro* metabolic stability of the compound across different species should already be known.
4. Major Clearance Mechanism in vivo: The major elimination pathways *in vivo* should be understood. Significant *in vivo* CL in one species may translate to other species, assuming that the *in vitro* correlation has been established. This could set the stage for performing clinical studies with the deuterated drug to confirm whether the desired change is observed.

Deuterated Therapeutics

Deutetrabenazine: This deuterated drug was approved by the FDA in 2017 (Austedo, Fig. 2.12). The deuterated carbons reduces *O*-demethylation by CYP2D6, hence increasing plasma exposure by two-fold (Schneider et al. 2020).[4]

D_3-Nevirapine (NVP): This deuterated compound lowers skin sensitization in rats by lowering CYP-mediated formation of 12-hydroxy-NVP, which undergoes further bioactivation via sulfation. (Fig. 2.12; Heck et al. 2020).

Deuterated carbazeran: In vitro, the KIE for aldehyde oxidase is 5 in multiple species, but the value is lower in hepatocytes due to competing glucuronidation (Kaye et al. 2009). In guinea pigs, deuterated carbazeran's KIE translates to an *AUC* increase of 22-fold for oral administration and six-fold for intravenous.

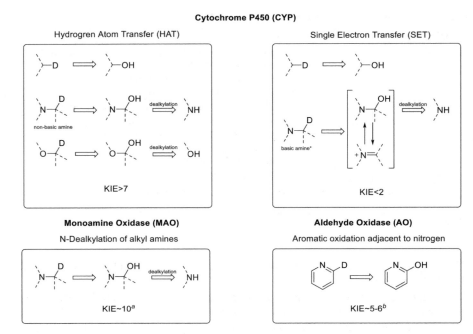

Fig. 2.11 Relevant drug metabolizing enzymes and their typical metabolic reactions that utilize kinetic isotope effects. ([a] Gaweska and Fitzpatrick 2011; [b]Sharma et al. 2012)

2.4.5 Peptides and Macrocyclic Peptides

Peptides are a unique group of molecules with distinct advantages that can engage targets not easily accessible by small molecules. Peptides are composed of between 2 to 50 amino acids and can be synthesized chemically (a chain that consists of 50 or more amino acids is considered a protein). Peptide therapeutics cover a broad spectrum of diseases such as metabolic diseases, endocrinology, cardiovascular conditions, gastroenterology, bone diseases, dermatology and sexual dysfunction. Many marketed peptide drugs have extracellular targets. Interest in this modality has increased recently with the advent of advanced technologies and improved understanding, in particular in the area of disrupting intracellular protein-protein interactions. Between 2015 and 2019, the FDA approved 13 peptides (Table 2.10), representing about 7% of the total number of 208 drugs (150 new chemical entities and 58 biologics; Torre and de la Albericio 2020).

Despite the advantages, there are major challenges to peptide drug development such as their low membrane permeability and poor *in vivo* metabolic stability, both of which lead to low systemic exposure, especially for oral peptide drugs. Hence, the major (~70%) administration route for peptide drugs is via injection.

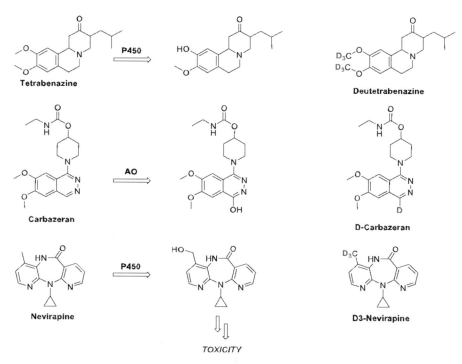

Fig. 2.12 The deuteration of tetrabenazine (Schneider et al. 2020), carbazeran (Sharma et al. 2012) and nevirapine, leading to improved metabolic stability

Modifications used to improve the drug-like properties of peptides can be seen in Fig. 2.13.

Strategies to Improve the Metabolic Stability of Peptides

1. *Side chain modification:* β-/D-amino acids have been used as substitutions to protect peptides from protease degradation. For example, Trulance® contains almost exclusively D-amino acids. Other side-chain functionality-modifying strategies yield peptidic molecules called peptidomimetics such as indinavir (Fig. 2.14). Azapeptides are peptidomimetics in which the α-carbon(s) of one or more amino acid residues are substituted by nitrogen (Chingle et al. 2017).
2. *Backbone modification:* α-Methylation and N-methylation are widely used backbone modifications. Peptoids are oligomers based on a polyglycine backbone in which the side chains are appended to the amide nitrogen (poly-N-substituted glycines) (Saini and Verma 2017).
3. *Cyclization:* A number of strategies exist for generating cyclized peptides. Cyclization can be achieved via an amide bond or other chemically stable bond such as disulfide, ether, thioether or lactone (e.g., teixobactin, Fig. 2.14). Head-to-tail cyclization results in a peptide bond between the original N- and C-termini. Examples of natural cyclic peptides in this category are gramicidin and tyrocidine with bactericidal activity, cyclosporin A (Fig. 2.14) with immunosuppres-

Table 2.10   FDA approved peptide drugs from 2015 to 2019

Year	Active ingredient (Trade name)	Indication	Features
2015	Insulin degludec (Tresiba®)	Diabetes	Modified insulin with an aa deletion and a hexadecanedioic acid via γ-Glu at the Lys (B29)
2015	Ixazomib (Ninlar®)	Multiple myeloma	N-Acylated, C-boronic acid dipeptide
2016	Adlyxin (Lixisenatide®)	Diabetes	44 aa GLP-1 peptide with (Lys)₆ at the C-terminal
2017	Abaloparatide (Tymlos®)	Osteoporosis	34 aa analog of parathyroid hormone-related protein
2017	Angiotensin II (Giapreza®)	Hypotension	Natural octapeptide
2017	Etelcalcetide (Parsabiv®)	Hyperparathyroidism	Ac-DCys-DAla-(DArg)₃-DAla-DArg-NH2 linked to L-Cys through a disulfide bridge
2017	Macimorelin (Macrilen®)	Growth hormone deficiency	Pseudotripeptide N-formylated
2017	Plecanatide (Trulance®)	Chronic idiopathic constipation	16 aa with two disulfides
2017	Semaglutide (Ozempic®)	Diabetes	GLP-1 peptide (31 aa in the chain) with hexadecanedioic acid via γ-Glu and mini PEG at Lys
2018	177Lu DOTA-TATE (Lutathera®)	Neuroendocrine tumors, theranostic	177Lu chelated by DOTA bound to Tyr3-octreotate
2019	68Ga DOTA-TOC	Neuroendocrine tumors, diagnostic	68Ga chelated by DOTA bound to Tyr3-octreotide
2019	Afamelanotide (Scenesse®)	Skin damage and pain	13 aa lineal peptide analog of α-MSH
2019	Bremelanotide (Vyleesi®)	Women hypoactive sexual desire	7 aa cyclic peptide analog of α-MSH

Torre and de la Albericio (2020)

sive activity, and vancomycin with antibacterial activity. Cyclization between side-chains, in particular, has proven effective at optimizing conformational stability for helical peptides, for example the stapled α–helical peptide ATSP-7041 (Chang et al. 2013).

4. *Capping the end groups:* This strategy protects termini against proteolysis and restricts conformational flexibility of peptides. C-terminal amidation or N-terminal acetylation are used for this purpose. Disulfide bridges can be used to cap the cysteine residue such as in Parasabiv® (etelcalcetide; Fig. 2.14). Disulfide bridges can also be formed between the cysteine pairs of the side chains to prevent random disulfide formation.

5. *Cystine knots:* The cystine knot motif has been applied to drug design as it exhibits thermal stability, chemical stability and proteolytic resistance. A cystine knot is a structural motif with a triple stranded antiparallel beta sheet linked by three

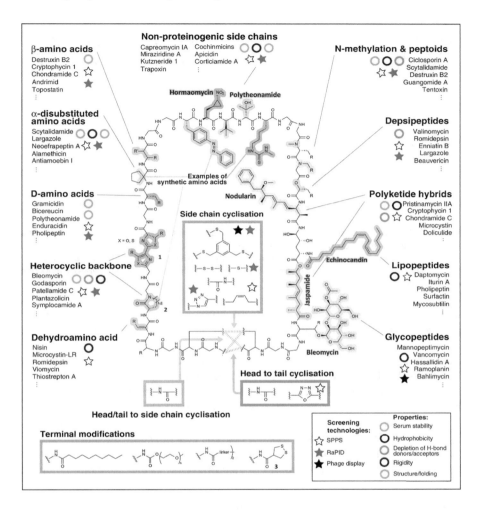

Fig. 2.13 Commonly used modifications to enhance peptide drug-like properties. (Walport et al. 2017; copyright obtained)

disulfide bonds, forming a knotted core. The hydrogen bonding interactions between the disulfide bonds of the motif and beta-sheet structures gives rise to highly efficient structure stabilization. Ziconotide is a synthetic 25-amino acid cystine knot peptide (Fig. 2.14) that is an N-type calcium channel blocker and inhibits the spinal signaling of pain.

Strategies to Improve the Intracellular Uptake of Peptides Improvement of membrane permeability or development of strategies that enhance intracellular uptake will facilitate peptide-based targeting of intracellular protein-protein interactions (PPi). Potential strategies include modulation of the hydrophobicity and elec-

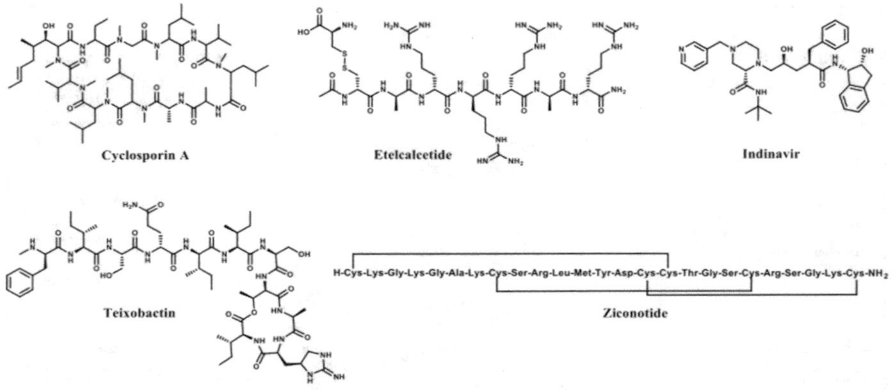

Fig. 2.14 Chemical structures of selected approved peptide drugs representing different features for enhancing drug-like properties. (Cyclosporin A (Sandimmune®): D-Ala, N-methylation and amide cyclization; Etelcalcetide (Parasabiv®): disulfide; Indinavir: peptidomimetics; ornithine and D-Phe; Teixobactin: 4 D-amino acids, Me-Phe, enduracididine, lactone cyclization; Ziconotide (Prialt®): cystine knots)

trostatic charges to improve passive permeability and conjugation of the bioactive peptide to a cell-penetrating peptide to facilitate its active transport (Lee et al. 2019).

Strategies to Improve the Pharmaceutical Properties of Peptides A number of liposome-based drug formulations have been used for drug delivery. Liposomes are vesicles composed of a bilayer (uni-lamellar) and/or a concentric series of multiple bilayers (multi-lamellar) separated by aqueous compartments formed by amphipathic molecules such as phospholipids that enclose a central aqueous compartment. In a liposome drug product, the drug substance is generally contained in liposomes. Typically, water soluble drugs are contained in the aqueous compartment(s) and hydrophobic drugs are contained in the lipid bilayer(s) of the liposomes (Bulbake et al. 2017).

Conjugation of peptides with non-biological materials (e.g., small molecules, metal chelates, polymers and hydrogels) is a promising approach to address the intrinsic drawbacks of the peptides. In particular, nanoparticles (NPs) have shown their potential to serve as conjugate scaffolds that not only improve the functionality of peptides but also implement abiotic characteristics, often resulting in synergistic effects (Jeong et al. 2018). Polymers or carbohydrates are also used for peptide conjugations. Examples of such polymers are polyethylene glycol (PEG), N-(2-hydroxypropyl)methacrylamide (HPMA), polysialic acid (PSA) and hydroxyethyl starch (HES). PEG protects against both enzyme degradation and reticuloendothelial uptake, which enhances a drug's pharmacodynamics and biodistribution. Examples of PEGylated drugs are aldesleukin, insulin lispro, PEGinterferon a-2a, pegfilgrastim, pegvisomant, insulin detemir, human growth hormone PLGA and bone morphogeneic protein 2 (Elzahhar et al. 2019).

Conjugation of peptides to larger plasma proteins such as albumin or IgG fragments can increase half-life and reduce renal clearance. For example, the FDA-approved drug, albiglutide, is a DPPIV-resistant GLP-1 dimer fused to human albumin. It has a half-life of 6–7 days, which enables weekly dosing for the treatment of type 2 diabetics (Di 2015).

2.4.6 Chimeric Degraders

Donglu Zhang

Chimeric degraders (also known as PROTAC = **PRO**teolysis **TA**rgeting **C**himera) modulate pharmacological activities through the degradation of target proteins instead of the inhibition of target activity (Fig. 2.4). These molecules have the potential to modulate targets that are not druggable by typical small-molecule compounds (Flanagan and Neklesa 2019; Pettersson and Crews 2019).

Two Structural Families

Mono-functional: This class of degrader targets a protein of interest to form a complex that initiates the protein-destruction machinery of the ubiquitin–proteasome system. These degraders have similar size and ADME properties as traditional small molecule drugs, but have often been discovered serendipitously (Pillow et al. 2020). Examples are GDC-0810, a selective estrogen receptor degrader, and immunomodulatory lenalidomide (Hanan et al. 2020).

Bi-functional: This class of degraders contains a ligand for the protein target of interest linked to a ligand for the ubiquitin-protein ligase (E3) (Pettersson and Crews 2019). Common E3 ligases are cereblon (CRBN), von Hippel Lindau tumor suppressor (VHL) and inhibitor of apoptosis proteins (XIAP) (Fig. 2.15). Target protein degradation requires several enzymatic steps that begins with the formation of the target-degrader-E3 ternary complex leading to the transfer of ubiquitins to the target protein by ubiquitin-activating enzymes (E1), ubiquitin-conjugating enzymes (E2) and E3. This tertiary complex brings the target protein and ubiquitination constituents into close spatial proximity. The ubiquitinated target protein is then recognized by the proteasome for degradation following dissociation of the ternary complex. The degrader molecule is then released to induce the next stoichiometric catalytic degradation of target protein molecules (Cromm and Crews 2017).

Because of the catalytic nature of bi-functional degraders, optimal PK profiles that support efficacy and safety are not essential. The bi-functional degraders have an event-driven pharmacokinetic profile instead of exposure-driven as is the case for most small molecule drugs. Degraders are large and flexible molecules and their physicochemical properties include high molecular weight (MW), high polar surface area (PSA), high number of rotatable bonds and poor solubility and permeability ('beyond Lipinski's rule of 5', bRo5 space). Consequently, the development of orally bioavailable degraders is a challenge and no formal DMPK strategies are in place to optimize these molecules for drug-like PK properties.

Tissue distribution and clearance are two key PK parameters that control the *in vivo* performance of a degrader drug. A degrader may never reach efficacious exposure at the target site if the compound is cleared too fast and/or is not distributed efficiently into the target tissue. Bi-functional degraders are expected to have limited membrane permeability and oral bioavailability based on the Ro5 established for small molecules. Consistently, low systemic exposure following oral or IV administration of several bi-functional degraders suggests that degaders are characterized by limited oral absorption and high clearance (Pillow et al. 2020). However, the orally dosed degrader, ARV-110, that was developed by Arvinas and entered clinical trials demonstrated that optimization of permeability is possible (Pettersson and Crews 2019).

The determination and optimization of many *in vitro* ADME and physicochemical properties like permeability, lipophilicity, pKa value(s) and protein binding is challenging for bifunctional degraders due to their large size and limited solubility. *In vitro* metabolic stability for degraders often does not predict *in vivo* clearance. Investigators have developed a trade-off approach to optimize ADME properties for degraders through emphasizing the importance of solubility as the key optimization parameter influencing oral absorption (Cantrill et al. 2020). Permeability of a degrader is unlikely to improve dramatically because of their large MW and flexible structure. Novel technologies are being developed to deliver these low permeability and low solubility degraders to their targets.[44] For example, conjugation of the BRD4 and ER degraders to engineered monoclonal antibodies provides a novel means of delivering these molecules to tumors *in vivo*. These conjugates appear to deliver efficient intracellular release of the degrader to support the biological activity.

2.4.7   Prodrugs

Prodrugs are drugs that have had a specific moiety altered to remove a liability such as high toxicity, low solubility, low permeability, short half-life and/or low chemical or metabolic stability (Table 2.11). The prodrugs themselves are inactive and need to be chemically or enzymatically converted to the active drug in the body.

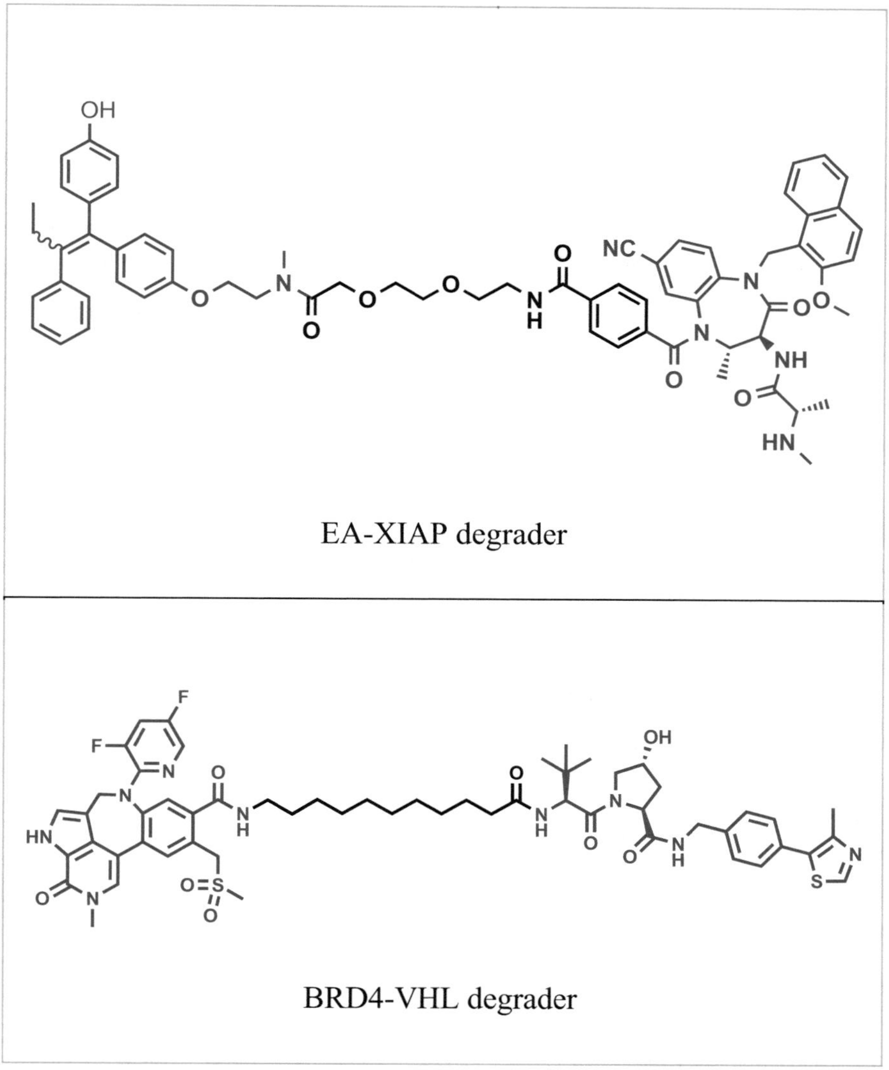

EA-XIAP degrader

BRD4-VHL degrader

Fig. 2.15   Structures of typical bi-functional degraders. (Pillow et al. 2020)

Table 2.11 Moieties used to enhance lipophilicity and solubility in prodrugs

Moiety	Alteration in prodrug	Enhanced properties	Release mechanism
-CO$_2$H	Ester, amide, carbonate, carbamate	Lipophilicity	Hydrolase
-OH	Ether	Lipophilicity	CYP
	Carbonate, carbomate, O-Mannich base	Lipophilicity	Hydrolase
	Phosphate	Solubility	Phosphatase
-NH (1°, 2°, 3°)	Amide, carbamate, N-Mannich base, oxime, imine	Lipophilicity	Hydrolase
	Phosphate	Solubility	Phosphatase
=O	Imine, oxime	Lipophilicity	CYP
-PO(OH)$_2$	Ester	Lipophilicity	Hydrolase
-SH	Thioether, thioester	Reactivity, lipophilicity	CYP, hydrolase

Case 2.3: Use of a Prodrug To Enhance Solubility

Chloramphenicol, an antibiotic, has poor solubility that makes it challenging to administer both by IV and oral administration. Two prodrugs are used that have improved solubility and undergo enzymatic hydrolytic conversion to chloramphenicol. • The succinate ester is used for IV administration. This prodrug is hydrolyzed in the blood with a conversion rate of 70%. The remaining amount is excreted as the prodrug in urine (Ambrose 1984). • The palmitate ester is used for oral administration and is hydrolyzed in the small intestine prior to absorption (Kramer et al. 1984).	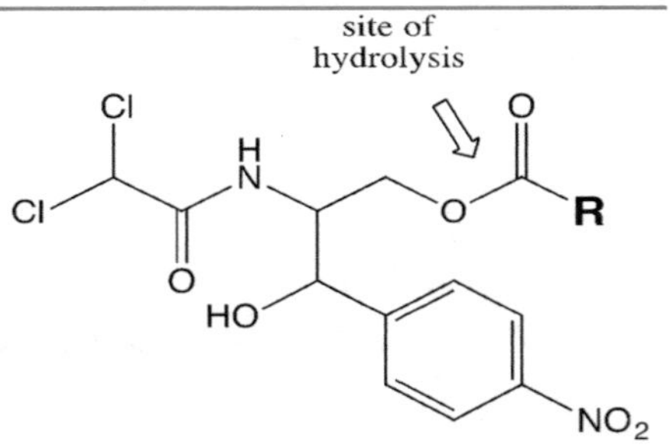 site of hydrolysis R = succinate for IV administration R = palmitate for oral administrations
Diazepam, an effective anxiolytic, has poor water solubility, which results in a slow rate of oral absorption. Avizafone is the prodrug and undergoes rapid hydrolysis by an aminopeptidase to give lysine and diazepam (Breton et al. 2006).	Avizafone

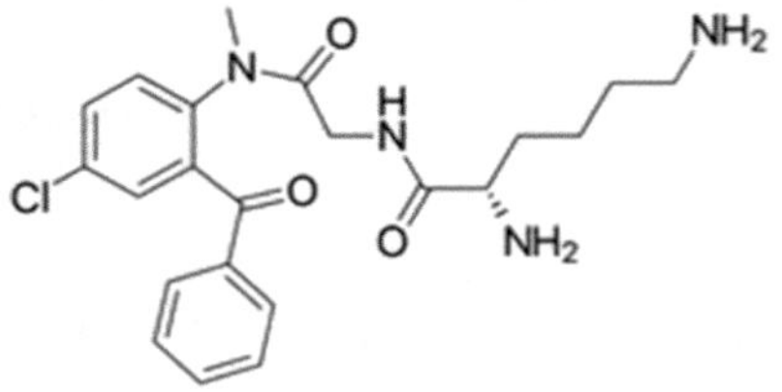

Case 2.4: Use of a Prodrug to Decrease First Pass Metabolism

Propranolol, a beta blocker for the treatment of high blood pressure, has low oral bioavailability due to high first pass metabolism by UGT that results in glucuronidation of the secondary alcohol. The hemisuccinate ester prevents direct glucuronidation and undergoes hydrolysis instead, resulting in a ten-fold increased AUC (Garceau et al. 1978).

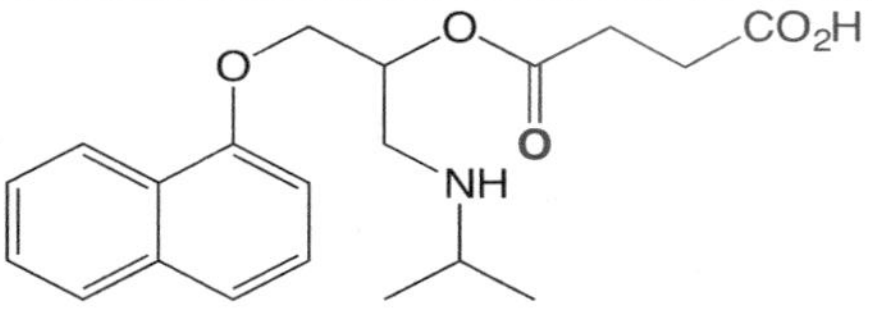

Succinate ester of propranolol

Case 2.5: Use of a Prodrug to Improve Permeability

O-Methoxy- and O-ethoxy-amidine analogues enhance permeability of amidine-containing molecules (Ansede et al. 2004).

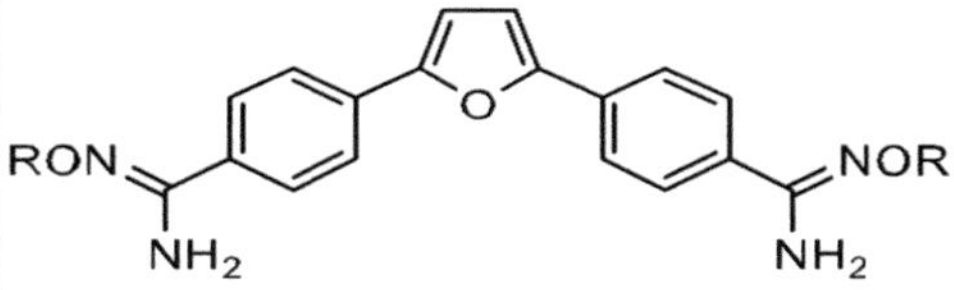

$R=CH_3$ or CH_2CH_3 metabolized to H

Case 2.6: Use of a Prodrug to Improve Oral Bioavailability by Uptake Transport

Levodopa is a prodrug of dopamine that is an LAT1 uptake transport substrate and can cross the blood–brain barrier. It is decarboxylated inside the cell to release dopamine, which has low permeability on its own. Thus, levodopa increases central nervous system dopamine concentrations for the treatment of Parkinson's disease.

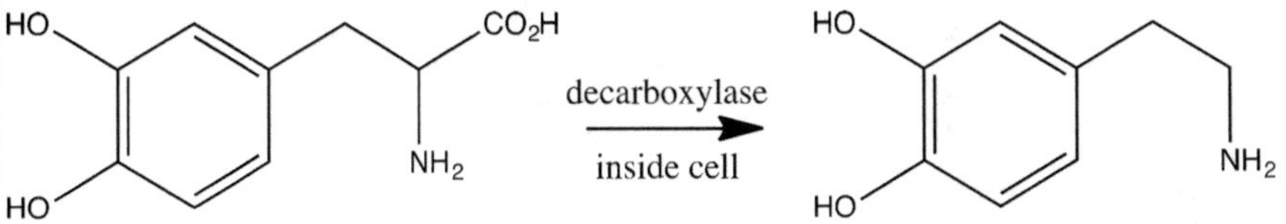

Levodopa

decarboxylase
inside cell

Dopamine

Human peptide transporter 1 (PEPT1) substrates

PEPT1 is an uptake transporter (high capacity, low affinity) that is primarily responsible for the absorption of dietary di- and tripeptides from the small intestine and can be used to improve the systemic exposure of a drug. Conjugation of the drug to form a prodrug with L-valyl ester or glycyl amide for example, improves bioavailability.

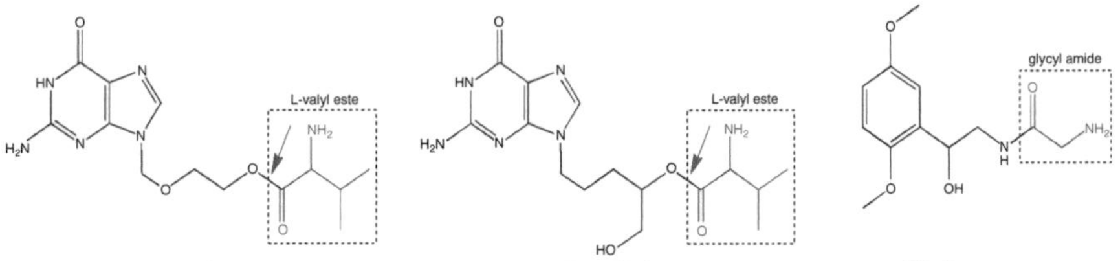

Valacyclovir

Valganciclovir

Midodrine

Case 2.7: Use of Prodrug to Increase Chemical Stability

Hetacillin is a prodrug of ampicillin (an antibiotic) that chemically releases acetone and the drug. The heterocyclic amine in hetacillin masks the chemically unstable primary amine in ampicillin, thus increasing the stability of ampicillin.

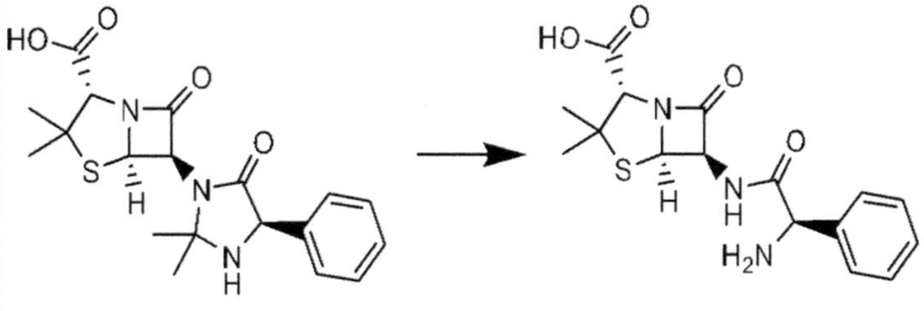

Hetacillin   Ampicillin

Case 2.8: Hydroxyamidine as a Prodrug and the Involvement of mARC

The basic nature of the amidine moiety in WX-UK1 (pKa ~11) diminishes absorption of the molecule. Upamstat is a hydroxyamidine prodrug that improves absorption and requires reduction by mitochondrial amidoxime reducing component (mARC) to form WX-UK1 (Froriep et al. 2013).

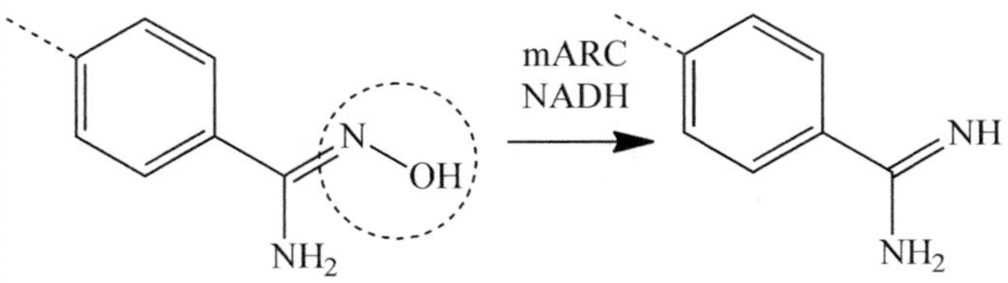

Upamostat WX-UK1

2.5   Metabolites as a Source of New Drugs

2.5.1   Secondary Metabolites from Natural Products

Natural products have been a traditional source for drug discovery. For example, morphine and codeine, the antibiotic penicillin, and the chemotherapeutic paclitaxel are all derived from natural products. However, natural product research requires intensive work for sample collection and the isolation and identification of the bioactive constituents amongst hundreds of compounds. In modern drug discovery, structural and ligand-based drug design introduced many *de novo* synthetic compounds as drug candidates. In addition to these intricately designed molecules, metabolites generated from xenobiotic compounds have provided another source for drug discovery and development.

2.5.2 Active Metabolites

An active metabolite is a metabolite with similar bioactivity as the parent molecule. Sometimes, active metabolites can exhibit more potent bioactivity, lower toxicity or better ADME properties than the parent molecule (Table 2.12). Consequently, the discovery of active metabolites opens a window to the evaluation and development of these metabolites as novel chemical entities.

In summary, numerous examples exist of active metabolites that have been or are being developed into drugs because of their advantages over the parent molecule, such as higher activity, improved ADME properties and/or enhanced toxicity profiles. Additionally, active metabolites generally have fewer liver enzyme interactions and are, therefore, a better option for patients with impaired liver function.

2.5.3 Targeted Approach for Active Metabolite Screening and Generation

Due to potential advantages and opportunities for active metabolites, some have incorporated assessment of major metabolites, especially when the PD response is higher than expected based on exposure. A targeted approach to generate and screen metabolites, such as the one shown in Fig. 2.16, offers unique time advantages in drug discovery. There are typically two ways to obtain the metabolites of interest: chemical synthesis and biosynthesis.

Chemical synthesis is traditionally the standard method of creating these metabolites. The metabolite of interest can be synthesized via the active pharmaceutical ingredient (API) or intermediates or through complete *de novo* routes, depending on the complexity of the molecule/metabolite. More recent approaches include biomimetic metalloprophyrin oxidations (BMO) as well as electrochemistry reactions. However, these methods often suffer inherently from requiring knowledge of the structure of the metabolite.

Biosynthesis, on the other hand, is a more straightforward process. Incubation of molecules with biomatrices such as liver fractions, engineered and recombinant CYPs, and microbes, leads to a "one-step" formation of metabolites (Shanu-Wilson et al. 2020). Major drawbacks of this approach are that the metabolites are synthesized in low quantities and are in a "dirty" matrix. However, with the advancement of modern instrumentation, a relatively "clean" metabolite of interest can be fractionated from bench-scale incubations (<10 mL) using LC-MS and analyzed

Case 2.9: Active Metabolites as Drugs

Morphine is an active metabolite of codeine by CYP2D6 mediated *O*-demethylation with five-fold higher activity and a longer duration of action (Goldsack et al. 1996). Morphine is further metabolized by UGT2B7 to morphine 6-glucuronide, which is an active metabolite with analgesic effect (Klimas and Mikus 2014).

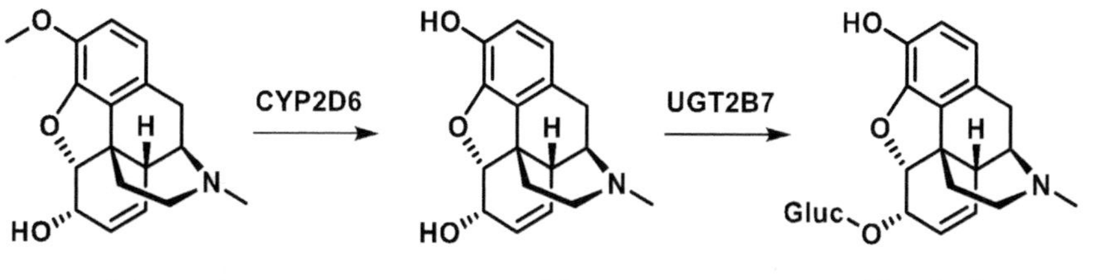

codeine → CYP2D6 → morphine → UGT2B7 → morphine-6-glucuronide

The tricyclic antidepressant amitriptyline was approved by the FDA in the 1960s and forms the active metabolite nortriptyline *via N*-demethylation. Nortriptyline is a more potent norepinephrine reuptake inhibitor than the parent drug with a five-fold lower Ki value towards the norepinephrine transporter (Vaishnavi et al. 2004).

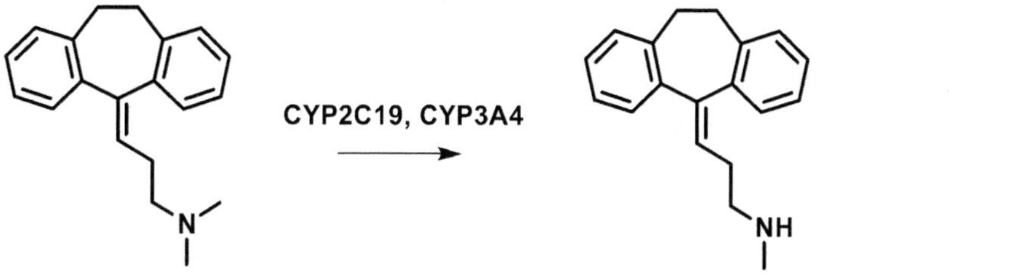

amitriptyline → CYP2C19, CYP3A4 → nortriptyline

Diazepam and subsequently its active metabolites nordazepam, temazepam and oxazepam were developed as the first-generation benzodiazepines, each with a different onset time and duration of action. Diazepam and nordazepam are long-acting (half-life >24 h) while temazepam and oxazepam are short-acting (half-life <12 h). Each of these metabolites undergoes further glucuronidation to form inactive metabolites

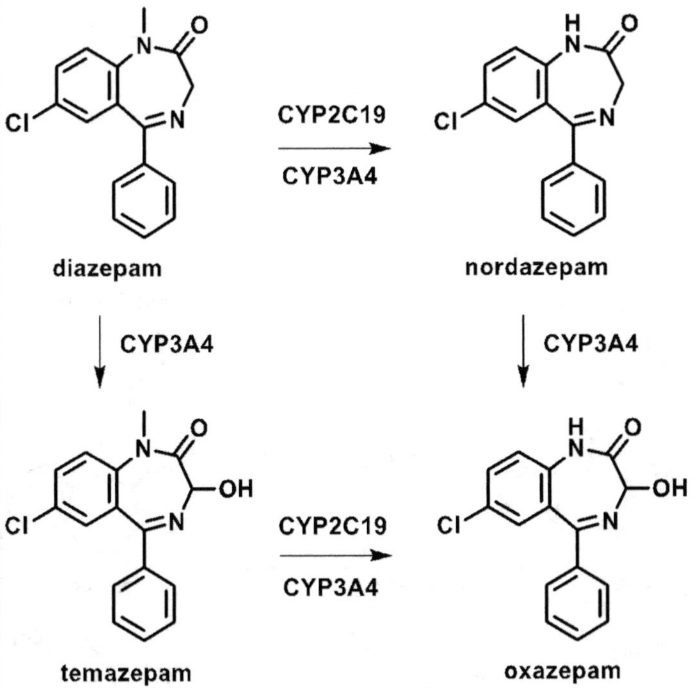

RDEA806 was designed as a non-nucleoside reverse-transcriptase inhibitor (NNRTI) for anti-HIV treatment. However, an unexpected dose-dependent decrease in serum uric acid levels was observed in the phase IIa study in HIV patients (Moyle et al. 2010). Its major metabolite, an amide hydrolysis product RDEA594, was found to be mainly responsible for this effect. This "active" metabolite was repurposed for development as a treatment of hyperuricemia. Both RDEA806 and RDEA594 went through phase I trials for this indication, but RDEA594 (lesinurad) showed much higher exposure and PD response. It was approved by the FDA in 2015.

RDEA806 → **RDEA594 (lesinurad)**

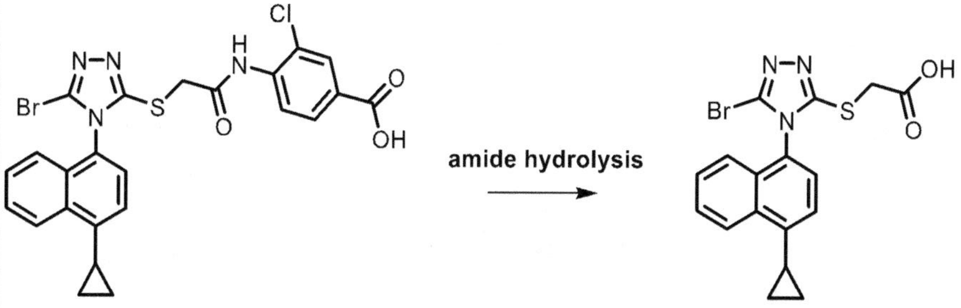

Case 2.10: Polymorphism of Drug Metabolizing Enzymes can Influence Drug Design

tamoxifen

CYP2D6

4-OH-tamoxifen/afimoxifene

CYP3A

CYP2D6

CYP3A

N-desmethyl-tamoxifen

endoxifen

tolterodine

CYP2D6

5-HMT

Esterases

fesoterodine

Tamoxifen is a first line treatment for ER+ breast cancer. It was later discovered that the pharmacodynamics of tamoxifen is a result of the CYP2D6-mediated formation of the metabolites 4-hydroxytamoxifen (afimoxifene) and 4-hydroxy-N-desmethyl-tamoxifen (endoxifen), both of which have a 100-fold higher activity than the parent (Desta et al. 2004). Consequently, the activity of CYP2D6, a polymorphic enzyme, plays a key role in driving *in vivo* efficacy of tamoxifen. Subsequent studies indicated a correlation between CYP2D6 activity and endoxifen concentration with the inhibition of breast cancer growth (Goetz et al. 2005; Schroth et al. 2009). The development of endoxifen as a drug in itself was particularly beneficial for patients with low-activity CYP2D6. To date, both endoxifen and afimoxifene have been extensively studied, and endoxifen was approved for expanded access by the FDA in 2019.

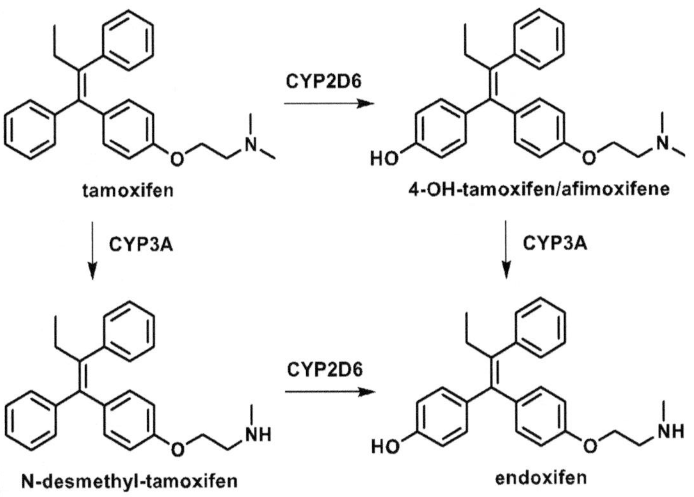

Tolterodine is an antimuscarinic drug to treat overactive bladder. Its active metabolite 5-hydroxymethyl tolterodine (5-HMT) is formed via CYP2D6. However, because 5-HMT has poor bioavailability, ester prodrugs, including fesoterodine, were designed with higher logD values to improve bioavailability. Additionally, fesoterodine forms 5-HMT via ubiquitous nonspecific esterases, and therefore exhibits CYP2D6 genotype-independent exposures (Malhotra et al. 2009).

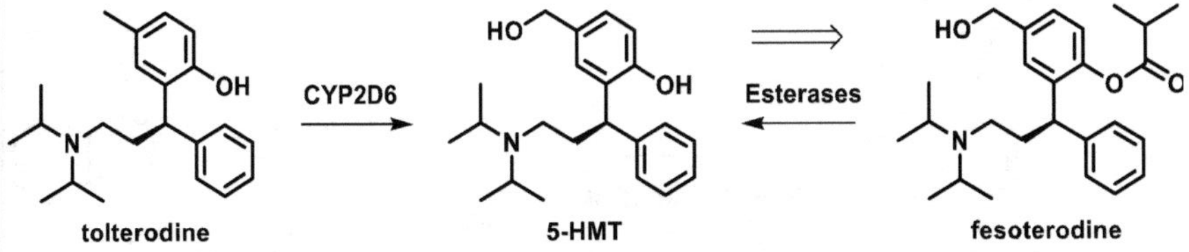

Case 2.11: Metabolites with Lower Toxicity

Hydroxyzine is a first generation diphenylmethylpiperazine antihistamine. Its major metabolite (cetirizine) in circulation is an oxidative metabolite formed via transformation of the terminal methoxy group to a carboxylate via aldehyde dehydrogenase. Cetirizine's basic piperazine nitrogen and acidic carboxylate make it a folded zwitterion with relatively high lipophilicity at physiological pH. The modified structure has a slower dissociation rate from the H_1 receptor and a less sedating side effect than hydroxyzine because of its lowered brain exposure. Cetirizine was developed as a second generation antihistamine. The third generation R-stereoisomer levocetirizine has higher selectivity with fewer side effects than the S-isomer (Chen 2008). This example also provides a strategy for limiting CNS penetration by modifying basic or acidic drugs to zwitterions.

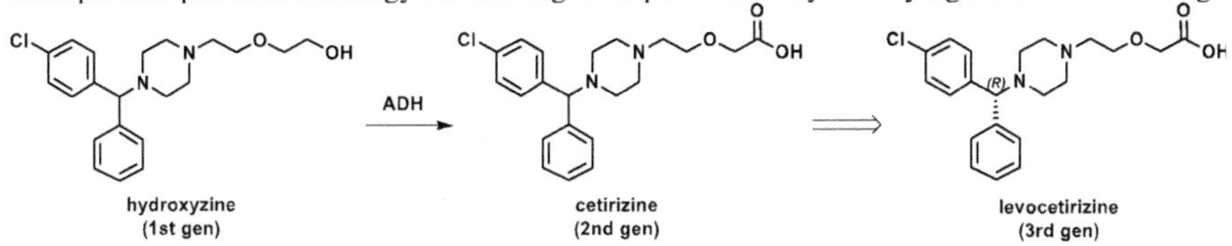

hydroxyzine
(1st gen)

cetirizine
(2nd gen)

levocetirizine
(3rd gen)

Fexofenadine is an active oxidative metabolite of terfenadine formed by CYP3A4 (Yun et al. 1993) and exhibits a similar potency for blocking the H_1 receptor. However, unlike terfenadine, fexofenadine does not exhibit cardiotoxicity due to hERG inhibition. Fexofenadine has, therefore, replaced terfenadine as a second generation anti-histamine.

terfenadine

fexofenadine

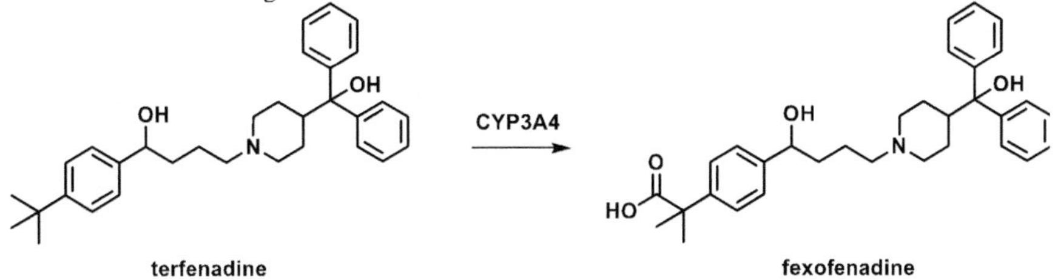

Table 2.12 Metabolites that provide advantages over or remove a liability from the parent molecule

Parent molecule	Metabolite drug (drug metabolizing enzymes)	Advantages over parent/problems solved
Tamoxifene	Endoxifene (CYP3A, 2D6)	Higher potency & less genetic variation
Tolterodine	Fesoterodine[a] (5-HMT via CYP2D6)	Less genetic variation
Amitriptyline	Nortriptyline (CYP2C19, 3A4)	Higher potency
Hydroxyzine	Cetirizine, levocetirizine (CYP2D6)	Fewer side effects
Terfenadine	Fexofenadine (CYP3A4)	Lower toxicity/fewer side effects
Diazepam	Nordazepam, temzepam, oxazepam (CYP2C19, 3A4)	Altered PK properties (elimination half-life)
Risperidone	Paliperidone (CYP2D6)	More available formulations
RDEA806	Lesinurad (hydrolase)	More predictable activity

[a]ester prodrug of metabolite 5-hydroxymethyl tolterodine (5-HMT)

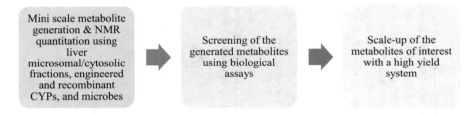

Fig. 2.16 Targeted metabolite lead diversification and SAR studies for a set of compounds can be efficiently achieved by following a three-step approach: multi-well plate metabolite screening using liver fractions and recombinant enzymes, screening of the generated metabolites, and scale-up of the selected active metabolites through a high yield system. (Lall et al. 2020; Stepan et al. 2018)

quantitatively and qualitatively with a high resolution NMR instrument coupled with a 1.7 mm cryo-probe (Walker et al. 2014). To obtain a metabolite standard for biological evaluation using quantitative 1D ^{1}H NMR, ^{1}H-^{1}H COSY, or multiplicity edited ^{1}H-^{13}C HSQC, a 1 mL incubation with 30 μM parent compound would be a sufficient starting point to obtain metabolites with a 10–20% turnover from the parent compound. Further, for more in-depth structural elucidation purpose, a 5–10 mL incubation would be needed to get good 2D experiments including ^{1}H-^{13}C HMBC.

References

Akamine T, Toyokawa G, Tagawa T, Seto T (2018) Spotlight on lorlatinib and its potential in the treatment of NSCLC: the evidence to date. Oncotargets Ther 11:5093–5101. https://doi.org/10.2147/ott.s165511

Alex A, Millan DS, Perez M et al (2011) Intramolecular hydrogen bonding to improve membrane permeability and absorption in beyond rule of five chemical space. Med Chem Commun 2:669–674

Ambrose PJ (1984) Clinical pharmacokinetics of chloramphenicol and chloramphenicol succinate. Clin Pharmacokinet 9(3):222–238. https://doi.org/10.2165/00003088-198409030-00004

Ansede JH, Anbazhagan M, Brun R, Easterbrook JD, Hall JE, Boykin DW (2004) O-Alkoxyamidine prodrugs of furamidine: in vitro transport and microsomal metabolism as indicators of in vivo efficacy in a mouse model of trypanosoma Brucei Rhodesiense infection. J Med Chem 47(17):4335–4338. https://doi.org/10.1021/jm030604o

Baillie TA (2016) Targeted covalent inhibitors for drug design. Angewandte Chemie Int Ed 55(43):13408–13421. https://doi.org/10.1002/anie.201601091

Bhhatarai B, Walters WP, Hop CECA et al (2019) Opportunities and challenges using artificial intelligence in ADME/Tox. Nature Mater 18(5):418–422

Breton D, Buret D, Mendes-Oustric AC, Chaimbault P, Lafosse M, Clair P (2006) LC–UV and LC–MS evaluation of stress degradation behaviour of avizafone. J Pharmaceut Biomed 41(4):1274–1279. https://doi.org/10.1016/j.jpba.2006.03.025

Broccatelli F, Wright M, Hop CECA (2019) Strategies to optimize drug half-life in lead candidate identification. Expert Opin Drug Discov 14(3):221–230

Brown DG, Wobst HJ (2021) A decade of FDA-approved drugs (2010–2019): trends and future directions. J Med Chem 64:2312–2338

Bulbake U, Doppalapudi S, Kommineni N, Khan W (2017) Liposomal formulations in clinical use: an updated review. Pharm 9(2):12. https://doi.org/10.3390/pharmaceutics9020012

Cantrill C, Chaturvedi P, Rynn C, Schaffland JP, Walter I, Wittwer MB (2020) Fundamental aspects of DMPK optimization of targeted protein degraders. Drug Discov Today 25(6):969–982. https://doi.org/10.1016/j.drudis.2020.03.012

Chang YS, Graves B, Guerlavais V et al (2013) Stapled A–helical peptide drug development: A potent dual inhibitor of MDM2 and MDMX for P53-dependent cancer therapy. Proc National Acad Sci 110(36):E3445–E3454. https://doi.org/10.1073/pnas.1303002110

Chankhamjon P, Javdan B, Lopez J, Hull R, Chatterjee S, Donia MS (2019) Systematic mapping of drug metabolism by the human gut microbiome. Biorxiv 538215. https://doi.org/10.1101/538215

Chen C (2008) Physicochemical, pharmacological and pharmacokinetic properties of the zwitterionic antihistamines cetirizine and levocetirizine. Curr Med Chem 15(21):2173–2191. https://doi.org/10.2174/092986708785747625

Chingle R, Proulx C, Lubell WD (2017) Azapeptide synthesis methods for expanding side-chain diversity for biomedical applications. Accounts Chem Res 50(7):1541–1556. https://doi.org/10.1021/acs.accounts.7b00114

Choo E, Boggs J, Zhu C et al (2014) The role of lymphatic transport on the systemic bioavailability of the Bcl-2 protein family inhibitors navitoclax (ABT-263) and ABT-199. Drug Metab Dispos 42(2):207–212

Ciancetta A, Sabbadin D, Federico S, Spalluto G, Moro S (2015) Advances in computational techniques to study GPCR–ligand recognition. Trends Pharmacol Sci 36(12):878–890. https://doi.org/10.1016/j.tips.2015.08.006

Cromm PM, Crews CM (2017) Targeted protein degradation: From chemical biology to drug discovery. Cell Chem Biol 24(9):1181–1190. https://doi.org/10.1016/j.chembiol.2017.05.024

Daublain P, Feng K-I, Altman M et al (2017) Analyzing the potential root causes of variability of pharmacokinetics in preclinical species. Mol Pharm 14(5):1634–1645

Degoey DA, Chen HJ, Cox PB, Wendt MD (2018) Beyond the rule of 5: lessons learned from Abbvie's drugs and compound collection. J Med Chem 61(7):2636–2651

Desta Z, Ward BA, Soukhova NV, Flockhart DA (2004) Comprehensive evaluation of tamoxifen sequential biotransformation by the human cytochrome P450 system in vitro: prominent roles for CYP3A and CYP2D6. J Pharmacol Exp Ther 310(3):1062–1075. https://doi.org/10.1124/jpet.104.065607

Di L (2015) Strategic approaches to optimizing peptide ADME Pproperties. AAPS J 17(1):134–143. https://doi.org/10.1208/s12248-014-9687-3

Di Paolo JA, Huang T, Balazs M, Barbosa J, Barck KH, Bravo BJ, Carano RA, Darrow J, Davies DR, DeForge LE, Diehl L, Ferrando R, Gallion SL, Giannetti AM, Gribling P, Hurez V,

Hymowitz SG, Jones R, Kropf JE, Lee WP, Maciejewski PM, Mitchell SA, Rong H, Staker BL, Whitney JA, Yeh S, Young WB, Yu C, Zhang J, Reif K (2011) Currie KS (2011) specific Btk inhibition suppresses B cell- and myeloid cell-mediated arthritis. Nat Chem Biol 7(1):41–50. https://doi.org/10.1038/nchembio.481. Epub 2010 Nov 28

Di L, Feng B, Goosen TC, Lai Y, Steyn SJ, Varma MV, Obach RS (2013) A perspective on the prediction of drug pharmacokinetics and disposition in drug Research and Development. Drug Metab Dispos 41(12):1975–1993. https://doi.org/10.1124/dmd.113.054031

Doak BC, Over B, Giordanetto F, Kihlberg J (2014) Oral druggable space beyond the rule of 5: insights from drugs and clinical candidates. Chem Biol 21(9):1115–1142

Edmondson SD, Yang B, Fallan C (2019) Proteolysis targeting chimeras (PROTACs) in 'beyond rule-of-five' chemical space: recent progress and future challenges. Bioorg Med Chem Lett 29(13):1555–1564

El-Kattan AF, Varma MVS (2018) Navigating transporter sciences in pharmacokinetics characterization using extended clearance classification system (ECCS). Drug Metab Dispos 46(5):729–739. https://doi.org/10.1124/dmd.117.080044

Elzahhar P, Belal ASF, Elamrawy F, Helal NA, Nounou MI (2019) Pharmaceutical nanotechnology, basic protocols. Methods Mol Biology Clifton N J 2000:125–182. https://doi.org/10.1007/978-1-4939-9516-5_11

Flanagan JJ, Neklesa TK (2019) Targeting nuclear receptors with PROTAC degraders. Mol Cell Endocrinol 493:110452. https://doi.org/10.1016/j.mce.2019.110452

Froriep D, Clement B, Bittner F, Mendel RR, Reichmann D, Schmalix W, Havemeyer A (2013) Activation of the anti-cancer agent upamostat by the MARC enzyme system. Xenobiotica 43(9):780–784. https://doi.org/10.3109/00498254.2013.767481

Garceau Y, Davis I, Hasegawa J (1978) Plasma propranolol levels in beagle dogs after administration of propranolol hemisuccinate ester. J Pharm Sci 67(10):1360–1363. https://doi.org/10.1002/jps.2600671007

Gaweska H, Fitzpatrick PF (2011) Structures and mechanism of the monoamine oxidase family. Biomol Concepts 2(5):365–377. https://doi.org/10.1515/BMC.2011.030. PMID: 22022344; PMCID: PMC3197729

Gehringer M, Laufer SA (2018) Emerging and re-emerging warheads for targeted covalent inhibitors: applications in medicinal chemistry and chemical biology. J Med Chem 62(12):5673–5724. https://doi.org/10.1021/acs.jmedchem.8b01153

Ghose AK, Viswanadhan VN, Wendoloski JJ (1999) A knowledge-based approach in designing combinatorial or medicinal chemistry libraries for drug discovery. 1. A qualitative and quantitative characterization of known drug databases. J Comb Chem 1(1):55–68. https://doi.org/10.1021/cc9800071

Gleeson MP, Hersey A, Montanari D, Overington J (2011) Probing the links between *in vitro* potency, ADMET and physicochemical parameters. Nature Rev Drug Discov 10(3):197–208

Goetz MP, Rae JM, Suman VJ et al (2005) Pharmacogenetics of tamoxifen biotransformation is associated with clinical outcomes of efficacy and hot flashes. J Clin Oncol 23(36):9312–9318. https://doi.org/10.1200/jco.2005.03.3266

Goldsack C, Scuplak SM, Smith M (1996) A double-blind comparison of codeine and morphine for postoperative analgesia following intracranial surgery. Anaesthesia 51(11):1029–1032. https://doi.org/10.1111/j.1365-2044.1996.tb14997.x

Hanan EJ, Liang J, Wang X, Blake RA, Blaquiere N, Staben ST (2020) Monomeric targeted protein degraders. J Med Chem. https://doi.org/10.1021/acs.jmedchem.0c00093

Harbeson S, Morgan AJ, Liu JF et al (2017) Altering metabolic profiles of drugs by precision deuteration 2: Discovery of a deuterated analog of ivacaftor with differentiated pharmacokinetics for clinical development. J Pharmacol Exp Ther *362*(2):jpet.117.241497. https://doi.org/10.1124/jpet.117.241497

Harnor SJ, Brennan A, Cano C (2017) Targeting DNA-dependent protein kinase for cancer therapy. ChemMedChem 12(12):895–900. https://doi.org/10.1002/cmdc.201700143

Heck CJS, Seneviratne HK, Bumpus NN (2020) Twelfth-position Deuteration of Nevirapine reduces 12-Hydroxy-Nevirapine formation and Nevirapine-induced hepatocyte death. J Med Chem 63(12):6561–6574. https://doi.org/10.1021/acs.jmedchem.9b01990

Hughes JD, Blagg J, Price DA et al (2008) Physiochemical drug properties associated with in Vivo toxicological outcomes. Bioorg Med Chem Lett 18(17):4872–4875. https://doi.org/10.1016/j.bmcl.2008.07.071

Jansson-Löfmark R, Hjorth S, Gabrielsson J (2020) Does in vitro potency predict clinically efficacious concentrations? Clin Pharmacol Ther 108(2):298–305

Jeong W, Bu J, Kubiatowicz LJ et al (2018) Peptide–nanoparticle conjugates: a next generation of diagnostic and therapeutic platforms? Nano Convergence 5(1):38. https://doi.org/10.1186/s40580-018-0170-1

Johnson TW, Richardson PF, Bailey S et al (2014) Discovery of (10R)-7-Amino-12-Fluoro-2,10,16-Trimethyl-15-Oxo-10,15,16,17-Tetrahydro-2H-8,4-(Metheno)Pyrazolo[4,3-h] [2,5,11]-Benzoxadiazacyclotetradecine-3-Carbonitrile (PF-06463922), a Macrocyclic inhibitor of anaplastic lymphoma kinase (ALK) and c-ROS oncogene 1 (ROS1) with preclinical brain exposure and broad-Spectrum potency against ALK-resistant mutations. J Med Chem 57(11):4720–4744. https://doi.org/10.1021/jm500261q

Johnson K, Le H, Khojasteh SC (2020) Identification and quantification of drugs. Metabol Drug Metabol Enzymes Transport:439–460. https://doi.org/10.1016/b978-0-12-820018-6.00015-6

Kaye B, Rance DJ, Waring L (2009) Oxidative metabolism of Carbazeran in vitro by liver cytosol of baboon and man. Xenobiotica 15(3):237–242. https://doi.org/10.3109/00498258509045354

Klimas R, Mikus G (2014) Morphine-6-glucuronide is responsible for the analgesic effect after morphine administration: a quantitative review of morphine, Morphine-6-glucuronide, and Morphine-3-glucuronide. Bja Br J Anaesth 113(6):935–944. https://doi.org/10.1093/bja/aeu186

Kramer WG, Rensimer ER, Ericsson CD, Pickering LK (1984) Comparative bioavailability of intravenous and Oral chloramphenicol in adults. J Clin Pharmacol 24(4):181–186. https://doi.org/10.1002/j.1552-4604.1984.tb01828.x

Lagoutte R, Patouret R, Winssinger N (2017) Covalent inhibitors: an opportunity for rational target selectivity. Curr Opin Chem Biol 39:54–63. https://doi.org/10.1016/j.cbpa.2017.05.008

Lall MS, Bassyouni A, Bradow J, Brown M, Bundesmann M, Chen J, Ciszewski G, Hagen AE, Hyek D, Jenkinson S, Liu B, Obach RS, Pan S, Reilly U, Sach N, Smaltz DJ, Spracklin DK, Starr J, Wagenaar M, Walker GS (2020) Late-stage Lead diversification coupled with quantitative nuclear magnetic resonance spectroscopy to identify new structure–activity relationship vectors at Nanomole-scale synthesis: application to Loratadine, a human histamine H 1 receptor inverse agonist. J Med Chem 63(13):7268–7292. https://doi.org/10.1021/acs.jmedchem.0c00483

Lee AC-L, Harris JL, Khanna KK, Hong J-HA (2019) Comprehensive review on current advances in peptide drug development and design. Int J Mol Sci 20(10):2383. https://doi.org/10.3390/ijms20102383

Leeson PD, Davis AM (2004) Time-related differences in the physical property profiles of oral drugs. J Med Chem 47(25):6338–6348

Lipinski CA (2004) Lead- and drug-like compounds: the rule-of-five revolution. Drug Discov Today Technologies 1(4):337–341. https://doi.org/10.1016/j.ddtec.2004.11.007

Lipinski CA, Lombardo F, Dominy BW, Feeney PJ (1997) Experimental and computational approaches to estimate solubility and permeability in drug discovery and development settings. Adv Drug Deliver Rev 23(1–3):3–25. https://doi.org/10.1016/s0169-409x(96)00423-1

Malhotra B, Gandelman K, Sachse R, Wood N, Michel M (2009) The design and development of Fesoterodine as a prodrug of 5- Hydroxymethyl Tolterodine (5-HMT), the active metabolite of Tolterodine. Curr Med Chem 16(33):4481–4489. https://doi.org/10.2174/092986709789712835

Maurer TS, Smith D, Beaumont K, Di L (2020) Dose predictions for drug design. J Med Chem 63(12):6423–6435

Moyle G, Boffito M, Stoehr A et al (2010) Phase 2a randomized controlled trial of short-term activity, safety, and pharmacokinetics of a novel nonnucleoside reverse transcriptase inhibitor, RDEA806, in HIV-1-positive, antiretroviral-Naïve subjects. Antimicrob Agents Ch 54(8):3170–3178. https://doi.org/10.1128/aac.00268-10

Nguyen L, Scandinaro AL, Matsumoto RR (2017) Deuterated (D6)-dextromethorphan elicits antidepressant-like effects in mice. Pharmacol Biochem Be 161:30–37. https://doi.org/10.1016/j.pbb.2017.09.005

O'Brien Z, Moghaddam MF (2017) A systematic analysis of physicochemical and ADME properties of all small molecule kinase inhibitors approved by US FDA from January 2001 to October 2015. Curr Med Chem 24(29). https://doi.org/10.2174/0929867324666170523124441

Page KM (2016) Validation of early human dose prediction: a key metric for compound progression in drug discovery. Mol Pharm 13(2):609–620

Pajouhesh H, Lenz GR (2005) Medicinal chemical properties of successful central nervous system drugs. NeuroRx 2(4):541–553

Pettersson M, Crews CM (2019) PROteolysis TArgeting chimeras (PROTACs) — past, present and future. Drug Discov Today Technologies 31:15–27. https://doi.org/10.1016/j.ddtec.2019.01.002

Phillips DH, Potter GA, Horton MN et al (1994) Reduced genotoxicity of [D 5 -ethyl]-tamoxifen implicates α-hydroxylation of the ethyl group as a major pathway of tamoxifen activation to a liver carcinogen. Carcinogenesis 15(8):1487–1492. https://doi.org/10.1093/carcin/15.8.1487

Pillow TH, Adhikari P, Blake RA, Chen J, Rosario GD, Deshmukh G, Figueroa I, Gascoigne KE, Kamath AV, Kaufman S, Kleinheinz T, Kozak KR, Latifi B, Leipold DD, Li CS, Li R, Mulvihill MM, O'Donohue A, Rowntree RK, Sadowsky JD, Wai J, Wang X, Wu C, Xu Z, Yao H, Yu S, Zhang D, Zang R, Zhang H, Zhou H, Zhu X, Dragovich PS (2020) Antibody conjugation of a chimeric BET degrader enables in Vivo activity. ChemMedChem 15(1):17–25. https://doi.org/10.1002/cmdc.201900497

Richardson K, Cooper K, Marriott MS, Tarbit MH, Troke PF, Whittle PJ (1990) Discovery of fluconazole, a novel antifungal agent. Rev Infect Dis 12(Suppl 3):S267–S271. https://doi.org/10.1093/clinids/12.supplement_3.s267

Ritchie TJ, Macdonald SJF (2009) The impact of aromatic ring count on compound Developability – are too many aromatic rings a liability in drug design? Drug Discov Today 14(21–22):1011–1020. https://doi.org/10.1016/j.drudis.2009.07.014

Saini A, Verma G (2017) Nanostructures for novel therapy. Synthesis, characterization and applications. Micro and Nano Technologies:251–280. https://doi.org/10.1016/b978-0-323-46142-9.00010-4

Salem AH, Agarwal SK, Dunbar M et al (2016) Effect of low- and high-fat meals on the pharmacokinetics of venetoclax, a selective first-in-class BCL-2 inhibitor. J Clin Pharmacol 56(11):1355–1361

Schneider F, Erisson L, Beygi H et al (2018) Pharmacokinetics, metabolism and safety of deuterated L-DOPA (SD-1077)/carbidopa compared to L-DOPA/carbidopa following single Oral dose Administration in Healthy Subjects. Brit J Clin Pharmaco 84(10):2422–2432. https://doi.org/10.1111/bcp.13702

Schneider F, Bradbury M, Baillie TA et al (2020) Pharmacokinetic and metabolic profile of Deutetrabenazine (TEV-50717) compared with Tetrabenazine in healthy volunteers. Clin Transl Sci 13(4):707–717. https://doi.org/10.1111/cts.12754

Schroth W, Goetz MP, Hamann U et al (2009) Association between CYP2D6 polymorphisms and outcomes among women with early stage breast cancer treated with tamoxifen. JAMA 302(13):1429–1436. https://doi.org/10.1001/jama.2009.1420

Shanu-Wilson J, Evans L, Wrigley S, Steele J, Atherton J, Boer J (2020) Biotransformation: impact and application of metabolism in drug discovery. ACS Med Chem Lett 11:2087–2107. https://doi.org/10.1021/acsmedchemlett.0c00202

Sharma R, Strelevitz TJ, Gao H et al (2012) Deuterium isotope effects on drug pharmacokinetics. I System-Dependent Effects of Specific Deuteration with Aldehyde Oxidase Cleared Drugs Drug Metab Dispos 40(3):625–634. https://doi.org/10.1124/dmd.111.042770

Sharma AM, Klarskov K, Uetrecht J (2013) Nevirapine bioactivation and covalent binding in the skin. Chem Res Toxicol 26(3):410–421. https://doi.org/10.1021/tx3004938

Shultz MD (2019) Two decades under the influence of the rule of five and the changing properties of approved oral drugs. J Med Chem 62(4):1701–1714

Smith DA, Rowland M (2019) Intracellular and intraorgan concentrations of small molecule drugs: theory, uncertainties in infectious disease and oncology, and promise. Drug Metab Dispos 47(6):665–672

Sriram K, Insel PA (2018) GPCRs as targets for approved drugs: how many targets and how many drugs? Mol Pharmacol 93(4):251–258. https://doi.org/10.1124/mol.117.111062

Stepan AF, Tran TP, Helal CJ, Brown MS, Chang C, O'Connor RE, Vivo MD, Doran SD, Fisher EL, Jenkinson S, Karanian D, Kormos BL, Sharma R, Walker GS, Wright AS, Yang EX, Brodney MA, Wager TT, Verhoest PR, Obach RS (2018) Late-stage microsomal oxidation reduces drug–drug interaction and identifies phosphodiesterase 2A inhibitor PF-06815189. ACS Med Chem Lett 9(2):68–72. https://doi.org/10.1021/acsmedchemlett.7b00343

Teague SJ (2011) Learning lessons from drugs that have recently entered the market. Drug Discov Today 16(9–10):398–411

Thomsen W, Frazer J, Unett D (2005) Functional assays for screening GPCR targets. Curr Opin Biotech 16(6):655–665. https://doi.org/10.1016/j.copbio.2005.10.008

Torre BG, de la Albericio F (2020) Peptide therapeutics 2.0. Molecules 25(10):2293. https://doi.org/10.3390/molecules25102293

Uttamsingh V, Gallegos R, Liu JF et al (2015) Altering metabolic profiles of drugs by precision Deuteration: reducing mechanism-based inhibition of CYP2D6 by paroxetine. J Pharmacol Exp Ther 354(1):43–54. https://doi.org/10.1124/jpet.115.223768

Vaishnavi SN, Nemeroff CB, Plott SJ, Rao SG, Kranzler J, Owens MJ (2004) Milnacipran: a comparative analysis of human monoamine uptake and transporter binding affinity. Biol Psychiat 55(3):320–322. https://doi.org/10.1016/j.biopsych.2003.07.006

Varma MV, Steyn SJ, Allerton C, El-Kattan AF (2015) Predicting clearance mechanism in drug discovery: extended clearance classification system (ECCS). Pharm Res 32(12):3785–3802

Vaz RJ, Li Y, Metz M et al (2018) Decreasing the CYP2D6 contribution to metabolism of a CK1ε inhibitor. Bioorg Med Chem Lett 28(23–24):3681–3684

Veber DF, Johnson SR, Cheng H-Y et al (2002) Molecular properties that influence the Oral bioavailability of drug candidates. J Med Chem 45(12):2615–2623. https://doi.org/10.1021/jm020017n

Walker GS, Bauman JN, Ryder TF et al (2014) Biosynthesis of drug metabolites and quantitation using NMR spectroscopy for use in pharmacologic and drug metabolism studies. Drug Metab Dispos 42(10):1627–1639. https://doi.org/10.1124/dmd.114.059204

Walport LJ, Obexer R, Suga H (2017) Strategies for transitioning Macrocyclic peptides to cell-permeable drug leads. Curr Opin Biotech 48:242–250. https://doi.org/10.1016/j.copbio.2017.07.007

Wenlock MC, Austin RP, Barton P et al (2003) A comparison of physicochemical property profiles of development and marketed oral drugs. J Med Chem 46(7):1250–1256

Wu CY, Benet LZ (2005) Predicting drug disposition via application of BCS transport/elimination interplay and development of a biopharmaceutics drug disposition classification system. Pharm Res 22(1):11–23

Yun CH, Okerholm RA, Guengerich FP (1993) Oxidation of the antihistaminic drug Terfenadine in human liver Microsomes. Role of cytochrome P-450 3A(4) in N-Dealkylation and C-Hydroxylation.Page??

Zang R, Ma S, Wright M (2018) Drug metabolism and pharmacokinetics perspectives for covalent inhibitor drug development. Medicinal chemistry reviews 53, chapter 22. ACS Publication

Chapter 3
DMPK Lead Optimization

Contents

Abstract The optimization and discovery of small molecule drugs has evolved in the past decades. Since the mid-1990s, *in vitro* ADME assays have allowed for systematic optimization of molecules based on key ADME attributes. This has had a huge impact on the molecular design cycles: design, synthesis, assessment and re-design.

© Springer Nature Switzerland AG 2022
S. C. Khojasteh et al., *Discovery DMPK Quick Guide*,
https://doi.org/10.1007/978-3-031-10691-0_3

In this chapter, we discuss the strategies for optimization of small molecules during drug discovery and address various ADME liabilities that exist during small molecule optimization. We have included many examples to allow for dissecting the problems and complexities of a real world drug discovery.

Keywords Optimization · Drug properties · Pharmacokinetics · Drug metabolism · Permeability · Drug transport · Plasma protein binding · Reactive metabolites

Abbreviations

ABC	ATP-binding cassette transporters
ASBT	Ileal apical sodium/ bile acid co-transporter.
AUC	Area under the blood/plasma concentration-time profile
$AUC_{Extravascular}$	AUC following an extravascular dose (i.e. oral, subcutaneous, intraperitoneal)
AUC_{IV}	AUC following an intravenous dose
BCRP	Breast cancer resistance protein
BSEP	Bile-salt export pump
CL	Clearance
C_{max}	Highest or peak blood/plasma concentration
DME	Drug metabolizing enzymes
E	Extraction ratio
F	Bioavailability
f_u	Unbound fraction in blood/plasma
f_{uT}	Unbound fraction in tissue
HBA	Hydrogen bond acceptors
HBD	Hydrogen bond donors
LC	Liquid chromatography
LM	Large molecules
MATE	Multidrug and toxin extrusion protein
MCT	Monocarboxylic acid transporter
MRP	Multidrug resistance-associated protein
MS	Mass spectrometry
NM	New modalities
NTCP	Sodium/taurcholate co-transporting peptide
OAT	Organic anion transporter
OATP	Organic anion transporting polypeptides
OCT	Organic cation transporter
OCTN	Organic cation/ carnitine transporter
OSTα-OSTβ	Heteromeric organic solute transporter
PEPT	Peptide transporter
P-gp	P-glycoprotein
PPB	Plasma protein binding
SLC	Solute carrier transporters

SM	Small molecules
Q	Hepatic blood flow
V_d	Volume of distribution
$t_{1/2}$	Half-life
t_{max}	Time at which C_{max} occurs
URAT1	Urate transporter

Case Studies

Case	Topic	Molecules
3.1	Improving bioavailability: Hiding HBD	razaxaban and apaxaban
3.2	Isosteres with switching between transport and metabolism	Prostaglandin d2 (PGD2) inhibitor
3.3	CYP2C9 polymorphic metabolism	BMS-823778 and 11β-hydroxysteroid dehydrogenase-1 for Type 2 diabetes treatment.
3.4	Blocking CYP metabolism.	Tolbutamide, chloropropamide, celecoxib
3.5	Using 1-aminobenzotriazole (ABT) in drug discovery	Celecoxib & its CF_3 analog
3.6	Novel AO role in hydrolysis	GDC-0834 (BTK inhibitor)
3.7	AO contribution to (1) high clearance, (2) low bioavailability, and (3) renal toxicity	
3.8	FMO substrates	
3.9	Blocking mEH Metabolism.	Oxetanes
3.10	Species differences in N-glucuronidation formation	mTOR inhibitor
3.11	Isosteres for optimizing hydrolytic reactions	Ritonavir and procaine
3.12	Isosteres of replacing phenyl with fluoro-pyrazole for blood stability	
3.13	Changes that resulted in metabolic stability.	
3.14	Molecular matched pair for optimization of metabolic rates	
3.15	Isosteres of morpholine with lowering clearance.	Entospletinib & lanraplenib
3.16	Isosteres of phenyl to pyridine to improve solubility and metabolic stability	T-type calcium channels inhibitors
3.17	Type I And II binding of pyridine to CYP resulting in inhibition.	
3.18	Fluoro substitution resulted in removal of CYP3A4 time-dependent inhibitor.	
3.19	Moieties that can result in reactive metabolite formation.	
3.20	Removing reactive metabolite.	
3.21	Isosteres of aminothiazole to fix reactive metabolites formation.	
3.22	Use of metabolic switching to remove reactive metabolites.	
3.23	Mechanisms of bioactivation.	

3.1   Pharmacokinetics

Pharmacokinetics (PK) is a "tool" that provides a quantitative description of what the body does to a compound/drug that is administered. Processes such as absorption, distribution, metabolism and excretion are described by PK parameters. In the drug discovery area, an understanding of PK in animals allows for selection and advancement of drug candidates.

3.1.1   Basic PK Terminology

3.1.1.1   Basic PK Terminologies Are Described Below

Table 3.1 PK parameters units of measurements and calculations

Parameters	Unit (example)	Calculations (equation)
AUC	Concentration × time ($\mu g \times$ hour / mL)	
C_{max}	Concentration (μg/mL)	
t_{max}	Time (hours)	
F	Percentage	$$F = \frac{AUC_{Extravascular} \, / \, Dose_{Extravascular}}{AUC_{IV} \, / \, Dose_{IV}} \times 100 \qquad (3.1)$$
CL	Volume/time (mL/min)	$$CL = \frac{Dose}{AUC} \qquad (3.2)$$ $$CL_{total\,body} = CL_{liver} + CL_{renal} + CL_{other} \qquad (3.3)$$
V_d	Volume (L)	$$V_d = CL \times \frac{t_{1/2}}{0.693} \qquad (3.4)$$ $$V_d = V_p + V_T\left(\frac{f_u}{f_{uT}}\right) \qquad (3.5)$$ V_p and V_T: volume of plasma and tissue f_u and f_{uT}: unbound fraction in plasma and tissue
$t_{1/2}$	Time (hours)	$$t_{1/2} = \frac{V_d \times 0.693}{CL} \qquad (3.6)$$
R	No unit	$$R = \frac{C_{max}(ss)}{C_{max}} \qquad (3.8)$$ $$R = \frac{1}{1 - e^{-kT}} \qquad (3.9)$$ T (tau): the dosing interval

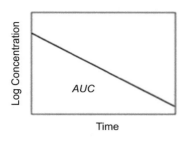
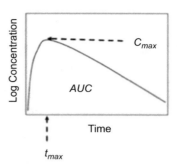

Fig. 3.1 Area under the concentration-time profile (*AUC*) following intravenous (left panel) or extravascular (right panel) administration. Highest or peak blood/plasma concentration (C_{max}) and time at which C_{max} occurs (t_{max}) are depicted following extravascular administration (right panel)

AUC Area under the concentration-time profile (*AUC*) is an important measurement of exposure and tends to be a more "robust" measurement of drug exposure than the measurement of drug concentrations in blood/plasma at a single timepoint. *AUC* can be assessed following intravenous or extravascular (e.g. oral, subcutaneous, intramuscular) drug administration (Fig. 3.1). Errors in drug concentration measurements at single timepoints generally have much less impact on *AUC*. Under linear conditions such as no saturating ADME processes, *AUC* increases proportionally with dose.

For a reasonable estimation of *AUC*, collection of plasma/blood samples should occur long enough such that the portion of the *AUC* that is extrapolated beyond the last measured concentration accounts for <30% of the *AUC* estimate.

C_{max}: Highest or peak blood/plasma concentration is an important measurement of exposure. Similar to *AUC*, C_{max} increases proportionally to dose under linear conditions. If performing non-compartmental analysis, this concentration is defined by the chosen sample collection times and the "true" C_{max} is not known. After intravenous dosing C_{max} usually occurs immediately following the completion of dosing.

t_{max}: The time at which C_{max} occurs is defined as the t_{max}. It is a measurement of the rate of extravascular absorption into the systemic circulation. Similar to C_{max}, when performing non-compartmental analysis, the t_{max} is defined by the chosen sample collection times and the "true" t_{max} is not known.

F: The bioavailability is the extent at which an extravascular (i.e. oral, subcutaneous, intraperitoneal, etc.) dose is available to the systemic circulation in relation to an intravenous dose (Eq. 3.1). Bioavailability is expressed as a percentage.

For oral dosing, a high bioavailability does not necessarily translate to great oral exposure. For compounds with very high clearance often you may observe high $F\%$ estimates due to a very low intravenous AUC. In addition, pharmacokinetic study designs often use high oral doses when compared to the intravenous dose. Since an oral dose is absorbed into the portal vein and must pass through the liver prior to entering the blood, saturation of hepatic first pass metabolism may occur. This scenario can result in a high F value that on occasion may be >100% (dose normalized) especially when high oral doses are given. Oral exposure of compounds should be ranked based upon both $F\%$ and oral AUC and interpreted in context of the oral dose given.

$$F = \frac{AUC_{Extravascular} \,/\, Dose_{Extravascular}}{AUC_{IV} \,/\, Dose_{IV}} \times 100 \tag{3.1}$$

CL: The volume of blood cleared of compound/drug per unit time and is usually determined following intravenous drug administration (Eq. 3.2). Clearances by various organs are additive. The total body clearance of a compound is a summation of the clearance contributions of various organs (Eq. 3.3).

Hepatic metabolism is the primary route of elimination for most compounds. A general assumption, although not always true, is that CL_{liver} (due to hepatic metabolism) is equal to $CL_{total\ body}$.

$$CL = \frac{Dose}{AUC} \tag{3.2}$$

$$CL_{total\ body} = CL_{liver} + CL_{renal} + CL_{other} \tag{3.3}$$

V_d: The volume of distribution is a proportionality constant relating half-life to clearance. V_d is related to clearance and half-life (Eq. 3.4). From a physiological point of view, V_d consists of the sum of the plasma volume and tissue volume (Eq. 3.5). The tissue volume is influenced by the degree of protein and tissue binding. For example, an increase in plasma protein binding in the absence of tissue binding changes will cause a decrease in f_u and a decrease in the volume of distribution.

$$V_d = CL \times \frac{t_{1/2}}{0.693} \tag{3.4}$$

$$V_d = V_p + V_T \left(\frac{f_u}{f_{uT}} \right) \tag{3.5}$$

V_p and V_t: volume of plasma and tissue.
f_u and f_{uT}: unbound fraction in plasma and tissue.

$t_{1/2}$: The time it takes for the amount of compound in the body to decrease to one half of the original amount is the half-life (Eq. 3.6). $t_{1/2}$ can be assessed after extravascular and intravenous administration but preferable following intravenous administration. An increase in V_d or a decrease in CL will cause an increase in $t_{1/2}$. It is important to note that CL and V_d are independent.

Estimation of the terminal half-life is sometimes influenced by the sensitivity of the bioanalytical assay. In cases where there is inadequate sensitivity and/ or low doses are administered, the terminal phase is not adequately characterized resulting in a much shorter than actual half-life estimate.

$$t_{1/2} = \frac{V_d \times 0.693}{CL} \tag{3.6}$$

3.1.2 PK Parameters and Drug Selection

From a perspective of drug candidate selection, compounds with moderate to low CL and longer half-lives, which leads to drug accumulation, are generally more desirable as these PK characteristics lead to lower doses. An estimate of V_d provides some context to how extensive the distribution of a drug candidate is and favorable characteristics of this PK parameter is generally determined on a case-by-case basis. For orally administered compounds, having a good drug exposure after oral dosing is a requirement and can be assessed by having good oral AUC and $F\%$. As oral PK parameters are formulation dependent, we discuss the interpretation of CL, V_d and half-life for the selection of drug candidates.

As many drugs are commonly cleared by the liver, hepatic CL often approximates total body clearance and can be categorized based upon its extraction ratio (E). The extraction ratio is the fraction of drug removed by the liver with each pass through the liver. For example, an E of 0.5 means that 50% of the drug passing through the liver is removed. For drugs cleared primarily by the liver, E can be approximated using the following equation with Q being hepatic blood flow (Eq. 3.7).

$$E = CL / Q \tag{3.7}$$

The classification of low, moderate, and high clearance based on extraction ratio is as follows:

Clearance	Extraction Ratio (E)
LOW	< 30% of hepatic blood flow
MODERATE	= 30–70% of hepatic blood flow
HIGH	> 70% of hepatic blood flow

Clearance Estimate is Higher than Hepatic Blood Flow

Categorization of CL as low, moderate and high based upon hepatic blood flow is important in the assessment of the pharmacokinetics of drugs and drug candidates. Most drugs are orally administered and compounds with low clearance result in better $F\%$ and oral exposure. Sometimes certain compounds will show clearances higher than hepatic blood flow. Three possible physiological reasons for this phenomenon include:

1. Compound is cleared by extrahepatic elimination pathways. Although hepatic metabolism is the most common route of drug elimination, it is not the only route.
2. Plasma clearance is often estimated rather than blood clearance (blood bioanalytical assays are much more difficult to perform than plasma assays). For compounds that preferentially distribute into red blood cells, the estimate of total body CL will be overestimated by the plasma clearance. This can be investigated by measuring the blood to plasma ratio of the compound of interest.
3. Compounds that are given intravenously that have extensive lung uptake can sometimes have clearance estimates that are greater than the cardiac output.

Finally, compound degradation in blood or plasma can result in an overestimation of clearance. In some cases, clearance estimates for compounds cleared by liver may be higher than hepatic blood flow because of instability in plasma/blood.

An estimate of the volume of distribution can provide context to how extensive the distribution of a drug is. However, favorable characteristics of volume of distribution is generally determined on a case-by-case basis. A comparison of a drug's volume of distribution to plasma or blood volume can provide some context as to how much a compound distributes out of plasma or blood and into tissues. For example, drugs that have V_d estimates much greater than plasma or blood volume will likely distribute extensively into tissues. Physiological parameters such as blood flows (Table 3.2) and volumes of various fluids and organs (Table 3.3) are used to aid in interpretation of clearance and volume of distribution estimates.

Table 3.2 Blood flows to various organs and tissues for mouse, rat, dog, monkey and human

BLOOD FLOWS in mL/min (mL/min/kg – assumes listed body weight)

Species (weight)	Mouse (0.02 kg)	Rat (0.25 kg)	Dog (10 kg)	Monkey (5 kg)	Human (70 kg)
Cardiac output	8.0 (400)	74 (296)	1200 (120)	1086 (217)	5600 (80)
Glomerular filtration rate (GFR)	0.28 (14)	1.3 (5.2)	61.3 (6.13)	10.4 (2.08)	125 (1.79)
TISSUES					
Adipose	–	0.4 (1.6)	35 (3.5)	20 (4.0)	260 (3.71)
Bone	–	13.5 (53.9)	–	–	218 (3.12)
Brain	0.46 (23)	1.3 (5.2)	45 (4.5)	72 (14.4)	700 (10.0)
Heart	0.28 (14)	3.9 (15.6)	54 (5.4)	60 (12.0)	240 (3.4)
Kidneys	1.30 (65)	9.2 (37)	216 (21.6)	138 (27.6)	1240 (17.7)
Liver (total)	1.8 (90)	13.8 (55.2)	309 (30.9)	218 (43.6)	1450 (20.7)
Hepatic artery	0.35 (18)	2.0 (8.0)	79 (7.9)	51 (10.2)	300 (4.29)
Portal vein	1.45 (73)	9.8 (39)	230 (23)	167 (33.4)	1150 (16.4)
Lung	0.070 (3.5)	2.3 (9.3)	106 (10.6)	–	–
Muscle	0.91 (46)	7.5 (30)	250 (25)	90 (18.0)	750 (10.7)
Skin	0.41 (21)	5.8 (23)	100 (10)	54 (10.8)	300 (4.3)
Thyroid	–	–	–	–	83.2 (1.19)

Davies and Morris (1993); Brown et al. (1997)

Table 3.3 Volumes of various body fluids and organs in mouse rat, dog, monkey and human

VOLUME in mL

Species (weight)	Mouse (0.02 kg)	Rat (0.25 kg)	Dog (10 kg)	Monkey (5 kg)	Human (70 kg)
Blood	1.7	13.5	900	367	5200
Plasma	1.0	7.8	515	224	3000
Total body water	14.5	167	6036	3465	42,000
Intracellular fluid	–	92.8	3276	2425	23,800
Extracellular fluid	–	74.2	2760	1040	18,200
Liver	1.3	19.6	480	135	1690
Brain	–	1.2	72	–	1450

Davies and Morris (1993)

3.1.2.1 Half-Life and Accumulation

The relationship between half-life and important PK parameters such as CL and V_d is illustrated in Eq. 3.6. However, half-life is also related to the amount of accumulation of drug after multiple doses. In Eq. 3.8, C_{max} is defined as the C_{max} after a single dose and $C_{max,ss}$ is the C_{max} after dosing to steady-state. R can also be defined similarly using trough concentrations after a single and at steady-state. Essentially, R is the factor that concentrations rise to after reaching steady-state following multiple doses. In Eq. 3.9, k is defined as the elimination rate constant (related to half-life as $t_{1/2} = 0.693/k$) and T (tau) is the dosing interval. Based on this equation, the longer the $t_{1/2}$, the more accumulation is anticipated following multiple doses to steady-state. The result will be lower doses required to reach target concentrations.

> **Effective Half-Life**
> There can be instances where the terminal half-life, despite being long, does not "help" in providing a lower dose. Specifically, advances in LC-MS/MS analysis has resulted in the ability to detect very low concentrations of a drug that may result in an estimation of a long terminal half-life. However, if these very low concentrations are far below therapeutic target concentrations at acceptable doses (eg. 1 mg/kg IV), the long terminal half-life contributes very little to providing a lower therapeutic dose. For the described situation, it may be more prudent to estimate an "effective" half-life using concentrations that are closer to therapeutic drug concentrations (Boxenbaum and Battle 1995).

$$R = \frac{C_{max}(ss)}{C_{max}} \tag{3.8}$$

$$R = \frac{1}{1 - e^{-kT}} \tag{3.9}$$

3.1.2.2 Oral Bioavailability

As the oral route of drug administration is the common route of administration, the oral bioavailability is an important compound property to consider when selecting drug candidates for further evaluation. As defined earlier, the calculation of oral bioavailability from PK studies is described by Eq. 3.1. Typically, the objective is to maximize the bioavailability by oral dosing. For an orally administered drug to enter the systemic circulation, the drug must be absorbed through the intestinal wall, enter the portal vein, pass through the liver, and enter the systemic circulation (see Fig. 3.2).

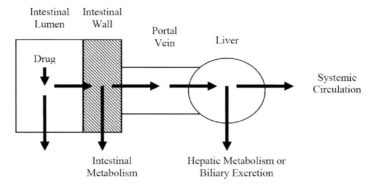

Fig. 3.2 Entry of drug into systemic circulation following oral delivery

As depicted in Fig. 3.2, metabolism can occur during passage through the intestinal wall and liver. Metabolism by the intestine and liver prior to reaching the systemic circulation is referred to as first-pass metabolism. Since bioavailability is a function of both absorption and first-pass metabolism of both the intestine and the liver, it can also be described by the following relationship:

$$F = F_a \times F_g \times F_h \tag{3.10}$$

F_a is the fraction absorbed from the intestine.
F_g is the fraction that escapes gut (intestinal) metabolism.
F_h is the fraction that escapes hepatic metabolism/elimination.

An alternative method of representing bioavailability in terms of extraction ratios is as follows:

$$F = F_a \times \left(1 - E_g\right) \times \left(1 - E_h\right) \tag{3.11}$$

E_g is the extraction ratio of the gut.
E_h is the extraction ratio of the liver.

Optimization of metabolism (and consequently E_g and E_h) is described in detail in other sections of this book. Oral absorption which influences F_a is dependent on the processes of dissolution and permeation across the intestinal wall.

The process of dissolution is the first step of the oral absorption process. Dissolution is an important factor that can influence both the rate and extent of oral absorption. The Noyes-Whitney equation (see Eq. 3.12) as shown below or modifications of it is commonly used to describe the dissolution of compounds.

$$Dissolution\ Rate = \frac{dX}{dt} = \frac{AD}{h}\left(S - \frac{X_{dissolved}}{V}\right) \tag{3.12}$$

X is the amount of solid.
$X_{dissolved}$ is the amount of dissolved drug.
A is the surface area available for dissolution.
D is the diffusion coefficient of the drug in the dissolution medium.
h is the thickness of the diffusion layer.
S is the solubility of the drug in relevant media.
V is the volume of the dissolution medium.

Based upon this equation, the main properties governing drug dissolution are:

1. The solubility of the drug in gastrointestinal fluid.
2. The surface area available for dissolution.
3. The concentration of the drug already in solution.

Based on EQ. 3.12, an increase in drug solubility would improve dissolution, and therefore, solubility is an important parameter to increase during medicinal chemistry optimization efforts. For specific drugs, solubility can be influenced by the solid state that it exists in. Crystalline forms of compound are less soluble than amorphous forms of the compound. Different crystalline forms (eg. polymorphs, salts, solvates) may also exhibit different solubilities. Physiological factors such as pH and bile acid concentrations can also influence compound solubility. Many basic and acidic drugs often exhibit pH dependent solubility profiles and therefore will have different solubilities in the stomach in comparison to the small intestine. Food intake can impact solubility by impacting stomach pH and also by increasing the concentration of bile acids.

Another parameter that improves dissolution is the surface area available for dissolution (A). The surface area for dissolution is directly correlated with particle size and shape. Dissolution rate can also be influenced by factors such as the wettability of the solid drug. Milling processes are often performed on solid drugs in order to decrease particle size and improve solid drug dissolution.

The next step of the oral absorption process is permeation across the intestinal wall. The permeation rate is governed by the following equation (EQ. 3.13):

$$Permeation\ Rate = \frac{dX_{dissolved}}{dt} = P_{eff} \times SA \times \Delta C \tag{3.13}$$

P_{eff} is the effective permeability of the drug to the intestinal membrane.
SA is the surface area available for intestinal permeation.
ΔC is the concentration gradient across the intestinal membrane.

As can be concluded from EQ. 3.13, improvements in solubility can also improve permeability by increasing ΔC. In drug discovery, permeability is often assessed during the drug discovery optimization phase using *in vitro* models such as Caco-2 or MDCK cells.

Assessments of oral bioavailability is often one of the primary reasons for running *in vivo* pharmacokinetic studies.

Pentagastrin Pretreated Dogs as a Model for Human Oral Absorption
Pentagastrin pretreated dogs are a preclinical *in vivo* model that have been used to assess pH-dependent and food effects on oral absorption. Specific to food effects, dogs exhibit a high variability in their stomach pH. Pentagastrin treatment helps to lower basal stomach pH in dogs and in addition reduces variability in stomach pH. Lentz et al. (2007), validated this model using a set of nine compounds with known propensities for human food effect.

Case 3.1: Improving Bioavailability: Hiding HBD

Oral bioavailability enhances placement of nitrogen in pyridine (Stearns et al. 2002). 2-Pyridine nitrogen atom hydrogen bond (HB) with the benzylic alcohol to enhance bioavailability.

Y	X	%F	
		Rat	Monkey
N	CH	17	4
CH	N	30	23

SN429 was pyrazole-based FXa inhibitor. The benzamidine coordinating with Asp189 that resulted in high potency (13 pM) but due to its charge and HBD it has poor permeability. In the evolution of this molecule razaxaban (190 pM) and finally apixaban (80 pM) were discovered that were not as potent but allowed for more appropriate ADME properties such as adequate permeability. The bicyclic pyrazole template in apixaban allowed for introduction of *para*-methoxyphenyl (Wong et al. 2011).

Target: Orally bioavailable factor Xa inhibitor.

SN429   Razaxaban   Apaxaban

3.1.2.3 Animal Selection for Preclinical Studies

Early PK studies are often conducted in common preclinical species such as mouse, rat, dog, or monkey. However, some thought should be placed based on what is known about metabolism and other clearance routes of the compound itself or its analogs in each preclinical species and the similarity to humans. Utilization of metabolism information for preclinical species selection can be illustrated in the following example. Shown in Fig. 3.3 are two plots examining correlation between microsomal intrinsic clearance (CL_{int}) in two preclinical species (dog and rat) versus human for a series of chemically similar compounds. For compounds from this "chemical series", the CL_{int} in rats correlates with the CL_{int} in humans. Assuming the compounds in this "chemical series" are primarily eliminated by metabolism, the rat would be the better preclinical species to perform PK studies with if the purpose is to select compounds with promising pharmacokinetics in humans. As metabolic stability studies are commonly performed prior to in vivo studies, this is an example where existing in vitro metabolism data can be leveraged in order to identify an appropriate preclinical species for pharmacokinetic screening.

Studies used to support preclinical efficacy or toxicity studies typically use the same compound form and formulation as was used in the respective studies.

Preclinical *in vivo* pharmacokinetics studies (see Sect. 6.3).

3.1.2.4 Higher Throughput PK Studies for Drug Selection

As *in vivo* PK evaluation still forms the back bone for drug candidate selection, study designs that increase the throughput of in vivo PK evaluation can be advantageous. These study designs are reliant on the selectivity provided by LC-MS/MS bioanalytical methods and include (Fig. 3.4):

- Cassette (or N-in-1) dosing
- Cassette Accelerated Rapid Rat Studies (CARRS) or Snapshot PK

These study designs when used properly can provide good in vivo data for the purposes of compound selection. It must be noted that these study designs should not be used to obtain "definitive" pharmacokinetics.

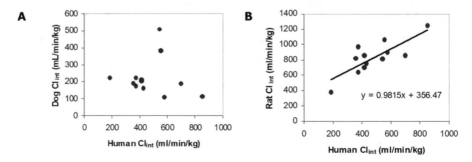

Fig. 3.3 Plots of (**a**) dog and (**b**) rat CL_{int} versus human CL_{int}

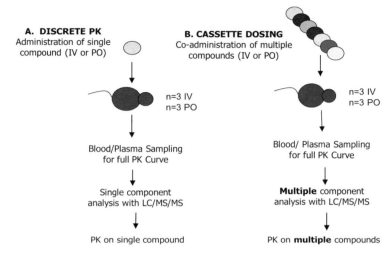

Fig. 3.4 (**a**) Discrete versus (**b**) Cassette (N-in-1) PK Study

Table 3.4 PROs and CONs of Cassette Dosing PK Studies

PROs	CONs
Higher throughput Reduction in animal and compound use Lowers cost of in vivo data (labor costs)	Bioanalytical challenges due to multicomponent analysis Increase in assay development time Potential assay interference by co-dosed compounds and their metabolites Reliability of PK data due to potential drug-drug interactions and protein binding interactions resulting from co-administration of many compounds

3.1.2.5 Cassette (or N-in-1) Dosing Studies

Cassette (or N-in-1) dosing studies involve the administration of typically 2–10 compounds formulated together to animals. An obvious advantage of this study design is that there is a large savings in animal use and personnel labor. For example, if 10 compounds are administered orally (N = 3) and intravenously (N = 3) as cassette formulations, the 6 animals used in the study can provide oral and IV PK information for 10 compounds. In discrete studies with the same number of animals for each route, 60 animals would be required to generate the same amount of PK information. As the multiple compounds are dosed at the same time, this study design relies heavily on the ability to analyze concentrations of more than one compound at the same time using LC-MS/MS. In addition to evaluation of systemic PK, cassette studies have even been successfully applied to evaluate CNS PK (Liu et al. 2012).

Obtaining useful PK data from a cassette dosing PK study requires careful attention to study design. The most common source of "not useful" PK data from cassette dosing studies is from drug-drug interactions resulting from the co-administration of many compounds at the same time (Table 3.4).

Common Errors When Performing Cassette Dosing Studies
- Dosing too high. For example, dosing 10 compounds at 10 mg/kg orally.
- Relying on cassette data as definitive PK data for the selection of candidate for higher investment toxicology evaluation.
- Not using a biological internal standard to monitor potential drug interactions caused by co-administration of multiple compounds.

3.1.2.6   Cassette Accelerated Rapid Rat Studies (Carrs) or Snapshot PK

Cassette accelerated rapid rat studies or snapshot PK are similar studies designs that serve to accelerate the acquisition of in vivo pharmacokinetic information. These study designs address concerns of potentially unreliable PK data that arise from co-administration of multiple compounds that can occur when performing *in vivo* PK studies. Cassette accelerated rapid rat studies or snapshot PK involve dosing of compounds discretely to rats (CARRS) or mice (CARRS & snapshot). The throughput for CARRS and snapshot PK is increased by reducing the number of animals used (N = 2), collecting only PO data, truncating the number of blood/plasma samples collected, and pooling blood/plasma samples from multiple compounds to save bioanalysis time. The tradeoff from these studies is that only partial PK parameters can be acquired to rank order compounds. Like cassette PK studies, they rely heavily on the ability to analyze concentrations of more than one compound at the same time using LC-MS/MS (Fig. 3.5).

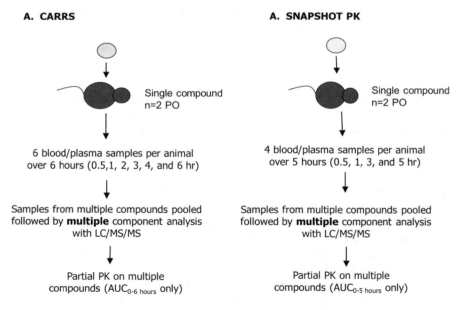

A. CARRS

Single compound
n=2 PO

6 blood/plasma samples per animal
over 6 hours (0.5,1, 2, 3, 4, and 6 hr)

Samples from multiple compounds pooled
followed by **multiple** component analysis
with LC/MS/MS

Partial PK on multiple
compounds ($AUC_{0-6\ hours}$ only)

A. SNAPSHOT PK

Single compound
n=2 PO

4 blood/plasma samples per animal
over 5 hours (0.5, 1, 3, and 5 hr)

Samples from multiple compounds pooled
followed by **multiple** component analysis
with LC/MS/MS

Partial PK on multiple
compounds ($AUC_{0-5\ hours}$ only)

Fig. 3.5 (**a**) Cassette accelerated rapid rat studies (CARRS) and (**b**) Snapshot PK study designs

The design of PK studies should be performed with an objective in mind so that adequate thought can be given to study design. There are examples in literature on the successful application of higher throughput in vivo study designs (Mei et al. 2006; Liu et al. 2008; He et al. 2008; Liu et al. 2012) so certain study designs are not necessarily better than others for purposes of compound selection.

What Are We Looking for When We Determine a Compound has Appropriate Pharmacokinetics?
Pharmacokinetic criteria for selection of compounds for further characterization often involves selecting compounds having the best combination of drug potency and favorable pharmacokinetics. As a general guideline, compounds with pharmacokinetic properties that allow for "higher" or "more sustained" systemic exposures are typically selected. For compounds that act *via* prolonged delayed pharmcodynamic effects, this general guideline may not apply, especially if toxicity is observed. For these compounds, it may be benefit to dose intermittently in order to avoid toxicities. Examples of this can be observed with classical chemotherapy where many agents have poor pharmacokinetics but are dosed at once weekly or longer intervals in order to avoid toxicities. Ultimately, the selection of compounds based on pharmacokinetics is highly dependent on what is required to elicit a therapeutically beneficial pharmacodynamics response.

3.2   Use of *In Silico* ADME Models in Drug Discovery

While attrition in drug discovery and development remains high, attrition due to poor human pharmacokinetics is relatively low with a recent analysis by AstraZeneca showing that about 76% of the human PK predictions fall within two-fold of the clinically observed PK (Morgan et al. 2018). Two important drivers of that are the availability of reliable human reagents (microsomes, hepatocytes, recombinant enzymes and transporters, etc.) and the ubiquitous availability of very sensitive and selective LC-MS equipment. These changes have allowed much earlier incorporation of ADME endpoints in drug discovery. Indeed, many companies routinely measure parameters such as metabolic stability in microsomes or hepatocytes, plasma protein binding and permeability in MDCK or other cells for many compounds synthesized in a project; these assays are usually very high up in the screening cascade. An added benefit is that data are generated for hundreds of compounds every week and these data are archived in the corporate database. For example, Genentech has data available for more than 100,000 compounds in mouse, rat, dog, cynomolgus monkey and human microsomes. These data serve two purposes: (1) provide insights **today** for a particular project and (2) enable the construction of *in silico* ADME models for any future project. The *in silico* ADME models can be used for any project at any moment in time and can be deployed **prior** to synthesis of compounds. The latter allows even earlier incorporation of ADME considerations and allows medicinal chemists to get an early read on the potential impact of design ideas to improve potency and selectivity on ADME endpoints. It is fully recognized that it is usually very hard to merge the complex potency, selectivity and ADME structure-activity/property relationships late in a project; doing so earlier in the life of a project may facilitate the optimization process greatly and enable finding a compound with the best balance of properties earlier and reduce the number of compounds to be synthesized. Overall, effective incorporation of *in silico* models offers the greatest advantages of all available new tools in ADME sciences.

In silico models have been around for more than 20 years and, in terms of being able to make reliable *in vitro* or *in vivo* predictions, most success has been achieved in the ADME field. Indeed, prediction of potency and selectivity, let alone *in vivo* toxicology, remains elusive although some progress is noticeable as will be described later on. Building *in silico* models begins with data gathering and curation. Most biopharma companies have a corporate database and, therefore, data gathering should be easy. However, the computational scientists still have to do a lot of curation, especially if the database contains data gathered using different assay conditions. Ideally, all data points have been gathered using the same set of experimental conditions. The latter is also the main reason why the use of data in public archives, such as PubChem and ChEMBL, is fraught with error. Obviously, a chemically diverse dataset is preferred for a global model. If the amount of data and the chemical diversity is limited, it may be possible to build a local model for a specific chemical series. The input data are the molecular structure and the *in vitro* ADME endpoint; models have been built for *in vivo* endpoints, such as clearance and volume of distribution, as well, but they are generally more complex. The dataset is split in two with the majority of the compounds in the training set and the rest (10–25%) in the test/validation set. Next, a large number of molecular descriptors are calculated for each compound in the training set, ranging from simple parameters such as molecular weight, log P, log D_{pH}, and TPSA to much more complex parameters reflecting the electronics and/or three-dimensional nature of the compounds. Those descriptors that most strongly correlate with the measured ADME endpoints are retained. (Deep neural networks can bypass this step and rely completely on the molecular structure.)

Multiple Approaches to Build Models Are Available:
- Regression methods (e.g. partial least squares)
- Bayesian methods
- Supervised learning methods such as decision tree (random forest (RF)) and support vector machine (SVM)
- Neural networks and, these days, deep neural networks (DNN)

A description of these methods is far beyond the scope of this book and specialized computational sciences literature is recommended. Finally, one or more models is built using those descriptors that correlate best with the measured parameter. (The number of descriptors should be kept limited to prevent over fitting.) Next, an independent validation data set is used to test each model and the most predictive model is deployed. Predictivity can be based on % true/false positive, true/false negative accuracy, sensitivity, specificity, correlation coefficient, etc. Models can be defined in most cases by their output: classification or numerical. The output of a classification method falls in a number of bins while for regression methods the output is numerical (although converting it to bins may be more appropriate to prevent over interpretation of the predictions). Ideally, the model also provides a measure of confidence in the prediction, which can be based on the presence (or lack thereof) of similar compounds in the training set.

It is important to use the output of the model appropriately – 'fit for purpose'. The goal is not a perfect prediction (even though that would be highly desirable). The latter would be an unrealistic expectation. The real goal is to **prioritize** molecules, ideally before they have been synthesized, and to improve the **odds** of success. An example is presented in Fig. 3.6. A microsomal metabolic stability model was built and the output was the predicted confidence in a compound being metabolically stable with >0.8 reflecting a very high confidence in being metabolically stable and < 0.2 characterizing a very low confidence in being metabolically stable (see Aliagas et al., 2015 for more details). It can be seen in the pie chart that more than 50% of the compounds predicted to be stable (>0.8) are indeed stable and less than 10% are unstable. On the other end, more than 90% of the compounds that are predicted to be unstable (<0.2) are indeed unstable. Thus, this model is very good at weeding out compounds that have very poor metabolic stability in microsomes. Depending on the specific status of a project, you can

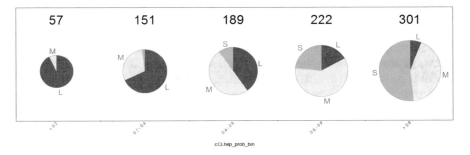

Fig. 3.6 Output of a Genentech microsomal metabolic stability model. The five bins reflect the predicted confidence in a compound being metabolically stable from low to high. The experimental results are presented in pie charts with green = stable, yellow = moderately stable and red = unstable in microsomes. The numbers above the pie charts represent the number of compounds in each bin for a particular project

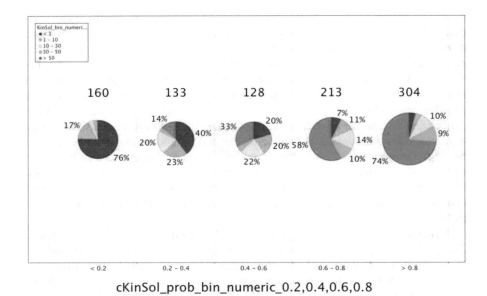

Fig. 3.7 Output of a Genentech solubility model. The bins reflect the predicted confidence in a compound having more than 30 μM kinetic solubility. The experimental results are presented in pie charts with dark green >50 μM, light green = 30–50 μM, yellow = 10–30 μM, orange = 1–10 μM and red <1 μM kinetic solubility. The numbers above the pie charts represent the number of compounds in each bin for a particular project

adjust the cutoff. For example, if you have many compounds that look promising from a potency, selectivity and ADME perspective, you can use a high cutoff, whereas you may want to be more generous in the early stages of a project when good leads are hard to come by. In this particular example, it is **essential** to confirm that microsomal metabolic stability is indeed the key determinant of *in vivo* clearance.

Models can be built for a wide range of physicochemical endpoints (lipophilicity, solubility, pK_a, etc.) and ADME endpoints (metabolic stability, permeability, efflux, plasma protein binding, etc.). The output of an *in silico* kinetic solubility model is presented in Fig. 3.7 and the interpretation is similar to that of the metabolic stability model. The bins reflect the confidence in kinetic solubility being more than 30 μM and the pie charts show the experimental data. It is clear that 83% (= 74 + 9%) of the high confidence predictions (>0.8) have indeed very good kinetic solubility. Moreover, it is very satisfying to see that the percentage of false negatives – compounds that are predicted to have poor solubility, but have high solubility in reality – is very low, <5%; it is the false negatives that medicinal chemists are usually most worried about.

Excellent examples of *in silico* ADME models and how these models impacted projects are presented in Lombardo et al. 2017, a cross-industry publication from the International Consortium for Innovation through Quality in Pharmaceutical Development. Commercial models, e.g. ADMET predictor (Simulations Plus), StarDrop (Optibrium) and SIVA (Simcyp), are available for quite a few ADME endpoints, but in house models are usually superior because of the more comprehensive data set available.

The use of Artificial Intelligence (AI) has accelerated progress (Bhhatarai et al. 2019) and models are available to predict potency and selectivity, albeit not in a quantitative fashion, but to prioritize molecules. It begs the question how close we are to a future where most optimization happens via *in silico* tools? Near term, augmented design may appear to offer the most promise with computational models proposing and filtering ideas and humans doing the final triage.

Attributes of Successful In Silico Models:
- Models should enable decision making, e.g. triage of synthetic efforts.
- Models should be fit for purpose; reducing risk and increasing the probability of the desired outcome should be the goal; being right all the time should not be the expectation.
- *In silico* models are ideally suited for idea generation.
- Use *in silico* models in concert with *in vitro* and *in vivo* data.
- Having the models is not sufficient; you need the right infrastructure, education and culture to succesfulle embed these models in drug discovery.
- Managing expectations; while models are not perfect, a validation excercise can inform the user of the value and limitations of a model.
- Models are the ultimate tool to bring to bring DMPK and medicinal chemistry closer together.

3.3 Isosteres

Isosteres are moieties that are used to replace another moiety to enhance drug properties. These changes are based on various properties from metabolism to permeability and solubility. The considerations for isosteres are from charge (pKa), size, conformation, polarizability, H-bond donor/acceptor, hydrophobicity, reactivity, stability and many other properties (Fig. 3.8). These are the basis of ADME scientists work closely with the medicinal chemists to contributes to drug design (Stepan et al. 2012).

Isosters of hydrogen atom				
Properties	**H**	**F**	**CL**	**CH₃**	**CF₃**
Van Der Waals Radius	1.2	1.3	1.8	2	2
Inductive Effect	-	3.1	2.7	0	2.8

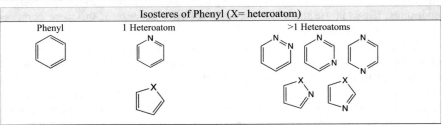

Isosteres of Phenyl (X= heteroatom)

Isosters of Carboxylic Acid		
Carboxylic acid pKa ~5	Tetrazole pKa 4.9	Sulfonamide EW=electron withdrawing

Even broader set of carboxylic acid isosters described by Lassalas (2016).

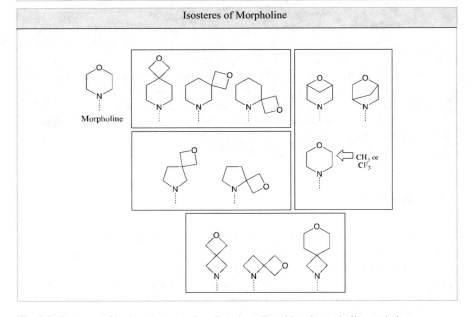

Isosteres of Morpholine

Fig. 3.8 Isosteres of hydrogen atom, phenyl, carboxylic acid and morpholine moieties

Case 3.2: Isosteres with Switching Between Transport and Metabolism

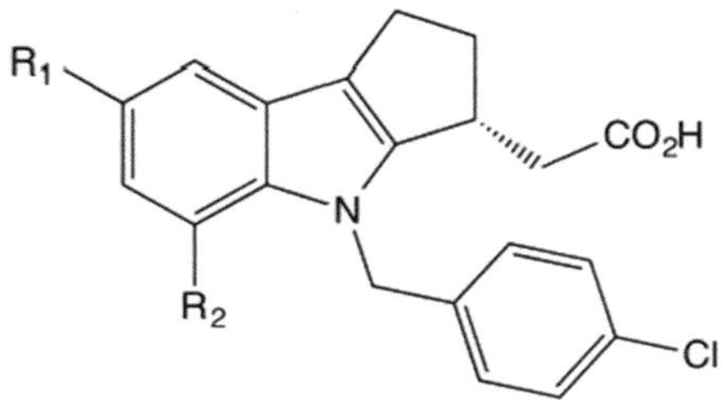

	R_1	R_2	Hepatocytes	In vivo plasma $t_{1/2}$ (h)	Concentration in bile (mM)
1	SO_2-CH_3	CO-CH_3	Stable	1.4	1.1
2	SO_2-CH_3	CHOH-CH_3	Stable	<1	3.9
3	F	CO-CH_3	Moderately stable	4	0.081

1. Both **1** and **2** are stable in rat hepatocytes but in vivo have relatively high clearance in vivo (short plasma half-life) (Sturino et al. 2007).
2. At the same time, they both had high concentration of the drug in the bile in mM range. This suggests that the in vivo clearance was not metabolic but rather dependent on efflux transport.
3. Replacing 7-methylsulfone with fluoro resulted in a less stable molecule in vitro, but improved the plasma half-life *in vivo* to 4 hours. This was explained with relatively low concentration of the drug in the bile. This suggests that the in vivo clearance was dependent on metabolism.

Target: Prostaglandin D2 (PGD2) inhibitor.

3.4 Metabolic Clearance Optimization

Clearance is a common term used for optimization of systemic exposure (Table 3.5). It is an additive property with combined metabolism and unchanged excretion. Metabolism is one of the major clearance pathways for most small molecule drugs followed by renal and biliary clearance (Smith et al. 2018).

The most used assays are focused on metabolism specially the one focused on hepatic and more specifically CYP metabolism followed by UGT (both liver microsomes and hepatocytes capture these). Models to predict renal and biliary excretion clearance is very limited and based on the current available models are not part of early screening tools.

Biliary Clearance Model
Sandwich-cultured hepatocyte (SCH) are in presence and absence of calcium buffer to modulate canalicular tight junctions are used to determine biliary clearance. B-CLEAR is an optimized model for this purpose (Brouwer et al. 2013). This model describes biliary excretion index and $CL_{b,int}$, allow for determining relatively contribution of hepatic drug transport in drug discovery. Rat SCH model allows for determining IVIVC and its relevance to human. This is only deployed where there is a high likelihood of hepatic transport involved.

Table 3.5 Major ADME challenges optimized during drug discovery process

Liability	ADME considerations	Endpoints
Short plasma half-life	High clearance	Metabolism (liver, extrahepatic) Non-metabolism (renal or biliary)
	Low volume of distribution (V_d)	Plasma protein binding Tissue binding
Low bioavailability (F)	Solubility	
	Permeability	Passive Drug transport
	Metabolism	GI, microbiome, intestine, liver
Drug-drug interactions (PK-based)	Inhibition	CYP, UGT, drug transport
	Induction	CYP, drug transport

For metabolic stability assays, there are several in vitro systems that are used for this purpose. They are typically examining the loss of parent drug over time. Timepoints of loss of parents are used for determining a half-life of the drug. For the hepatic assays half-life of parent drug disappearance, intrinsic clearance (CL_{int}) and predicted hepatic clearance (CL_{liver}) are calculated.

Extrahepatic CL
Theoretically the clearance parameters can also be derived for extrahepatic tissues, but it is more complex. For example, since CYP is mostly present in Clara cells in lung, if the whole lung tissue is examined for CYP metabolic rates, little to no turn over may be observed. However, at the cellular level the turn over per cell could be much higher. This is called tissue dilution and it is mainly due to the tissue architecture. The same could be said about the heterogenous distribution of the DME in tissues such as kidney, intestine, and others.

Beyond CYP
The experience of predictions beyond CYP is limited and not always consistent. In the discovery process one can examine the in vitro metabolism compared to in vitro clearance. If alignment is there for one species one could have a higher confidence for other species and most importantly human (Fan et al. 2016).

In Metabolism the Factors That Are Important Are:
- The contribution of metabolism to the total clearance.
- What type of reaction are involved? Types of reactions:

    Phase I: oxidation, reduction and hydrolysis.
    Phase II: conjugation

- What are the **drug metabolizing enzymes** (DME)? For this one needs to know (1) types of reactions, (2) subcellular locations, (3) cofactors, (4) organ distributions, (5) mechanisms of reactions, (6) known substrates and inhibitors.

By knowing these factors it allows for making structural modification to retain potency and yet removing the metabolic soft spot.

It is important to know the diversity of metabolic pathways that are possible. The scope of knowing the enzymes is based on the understanding of the biotransformation. Typically, but not always, oxidation by CYP is the first to be considered. This information is complemented based on in vivo understanding of metabolism. More routinely, liver is considering the major organ to examine for metabolism as it includes wide variety of drug metabolizing enzymes. This is followed by blood/plasma, intestine, kidney and lung.

Physicochemical properties Relationship to Metabolic Soft Spot
General physicochemical properties include charge state to lipophilicity (logP or logD), TPSA to hydrogen bond donors (HBD) and acceptors (HBA). These calculations are now a commonplace and it is important to make the comparison between molecules to further examine how these properties are changing during optimization (see Sect. 2.5). The specific structural properties in most cases drives the necessary changes in the metabolic clearance. This requires to have biotransformation information from the site of metabolism (soft spot) to the drug-metabolizing enzymes involved (Broccatelli et al. 2019).

Balancing Clearance Pathways
Having a molecule to have only one mode of clearance could be challenging. For example, if the molecule is only cleared through metabolism by CYP2D6 enzymes, then changes to the expression of this enzymes (as this enzyme is polymorphic) and differences between intra-subject variability will result in big changes in half-life of the drug in the body. In addition, there is a greater drug-drug interaction potential.

Polymorphic Metabolism
If certain polymorphic enzymes contribute to significant clearance of the compound, then there will be significant differences in clearance between poor and extensive metabolizers.

Genetic polymorphisms are stable variations (allele variants) of the gene that encodes a DME and are observed in at least 1% of a specific population. Genetic polymorphisms are designated by the symbol * followed by a number (for example, *CYP2D6*3*. Note that genes are italicized). The numbering scheme is based on when the variant was discovered. The wild type gene is designated as *1. Genotyping or phenotyping can be used for determining the metabolic capacity of polymorphic enzymes, which can result in changes in the pharmacokinetic properties of a drug.

The field of research that looks at the interaction between genetics and therapeutic drugs is called pharmacogenetics or pharmacogenomics.

For Caucasians, 1–3% are poor metabolizers (PMs) with respect to CYP2C9, 3–5% with respect to CYP2C19 and 5–10% with respect to CYP2D6.

Case 3.3: CYP2C9 Polymorphic metabolism

BMS-823778 major metabolite (M1) is generated by CYP2C9. Polymorphism of CYP2C9 result in poor metabolizer (PM) exhibited significantly higher plasma exposure of the drug (~five fold) than EM (Cheng et al. 2018). **Target:** 11β-hydroxysteroid dehydrogenase-1 for Type 2 diabetes treatment.	

BMS-823778
Arrow: site of CYP2C9 oxidation

3.4.1   Optimization Based on Drug Metabolism Enzymes

Drug metabolizing enzymes are diverse in function and reaction. Knowledge about these enzymes allow for developing strategies to overcome and modulate the rate and sites of metabolism (soft spot).

1. Cytochrome P450 (CYP or P450).
2. Aldehyde oxidase (AO)
3. Flavin containing monooxygenase (FMO).
4. Epoxide hydrolase (EH).
5. Uridine diphosphate glucuronosyltransferases (UGT).

3.4.1.1   Cytochrome P450 Enzymes (CYP or P450)

CYP or P450: Membrane-bound to the cytoplasmic side of the endoplasmic reticulum (ER).

Cofactor: Reduced Nicotinamide adenine dinucleotide phosphate (NADPH).

CYP nomenclature is based on the amino acid (aa) sequence. CYP**3A4**: **3** (family with >40% aa identity), **A** (subfamily with 40–70% aa identity), **4** (individual isoform in the subfamily with>70% aa identity).

CYP families that play a major role in the metabolism of drugs: CYP1, CYP2 and CYP3 (Tables 3.6, 3.7, and 3.8).

> **An orthologous form** of an enzyme is a similar gene product from the same evolutionary origin present in different species. Orthologous forms can be very similar, such as CYP1A2 in rat and human, or different, as in the case of CYP3A1 in rat and CYP3A4 in human. For this reason, substrate and inhibitor specificity between orthologous forms are never totally identical, and sometimes, they are very different.

Table 3.6 CYP isoforms and their abundance in the human liver (Rostami-Hodjegan and Tucker 2007) and intestine (Paine et al. 2006)

CYP isoform	Mean abundance in human liver pmol/mg (% total)	Mean abundance in human intestine pmol/mg (% total)	P450 Contribution to metabolism in marketed drugs (%)[a]
CYP1A1	Not detected	5.6 (7.4%)	
CYP1A2	37 (11%)		9%
CYP2A6	29 (8.6%)		
CYP2B6	7 (2.1%)		2%
CYP2C8	19 (5.7%)		
CYP2C9*	60 (18%)	8.4 (11%)	16%
CYP2C19*	9 (2.7%)	1.0 (1.3%)	12%
CYP2D6*	7 (2.1%)	0.5 (0.7%)	12%
CYP2E1	49 (15%)		2%
CYP2J2		0.9 (1.4%)	
CYP3A4	131 (40%)	43 (57%)	46%
CYP3A5		16 (21%)	

[a]The percent contribution of CYP isoforms to metabolism of the top 200 marketed drugs (Williams et al. 2004). *a polymorphic CYP isoform (see 'Genetic polymorphisms' below for percentages)

Table 3.7 Locations of CYP isoforms in humans plus factors influencing their expression

CYP isoform	Tissue	Factor
CYP1A1	Liver, lung, kidney, GI tract, skin, placenta	Nutrition, smoking, drugs, environment
CYP1B1	Liver, skin, kidney, prostate, mammary glands	Environment
CYP2A6	Liver, lung, nasal membrane	Drugs, environment, polymorphic
CYP2B6	GI tract, liver, lung	Drugs, environment
CYP2C	GI tract (small intestine mucosa), larynx, liver, lung	Drugs, polymorphic
CYP2D6	GI tract, liver	Polymorphic, not inducible (there was a report on corticosteroids that was retracted (Farooq et al. 2016),
CYP2E1	Liver, lung, placenta	Nutrition, environment, polymorphic?
CYP2F1	Liver, lung, placenta	
CYP2J2	Heart, intestine, liver	
CYP3A	GI tract, liver, lung, placenta, fetus, uterus, kidney	Nutrition, drugs, environment

GI gastrointestinal
Rendic and Carlo (2010)

Table 3.8 Typical characteristics of human CYP substrates

Isoform	Charge	Substrate Characteristics
CYP1A2	B, N	Planar polyaromatic, one hydrogen bond donor, may contain amines or amides
CYP2A6	B, N	Small size, non-planar, at least one aromatic ring
CYP2B6	B, N	Medium size, angular, 1–2 H-bond donors or acceptors
CYP2C8	A, N	Large size, elongated
CYP2C9	A	Medium size, 1–2 H-bond donors, lipophilic
CYP2C19	B	2–3 H-bond acceptors, moderately lipophilic
CYP2D6	B	Medium size, 5–7 Å distance between basic nitrogen and site of oxidation
CYP2E1	N	Small size, hydrophilic, relatively planar
CYP3A	B, A, N	Large size, lipophilic

Charge basic (B), acidic (A) or neutral (N) substrates

Case 3.4: Blocking CYP Metabolism

Tolbutamide is metabolized by mainly CYP2C9 at the benzylic methyl position. Substitution by chloro (**Chloropropamide**) has a longer human plasma half-life due to (1) blocking of the oxidation site and (2) the phenyl ring more electron deficient and hence less prone to CYP oxidation. (Xu et al. 2009).
Target: treatment of mellitus type 2 diabetes.

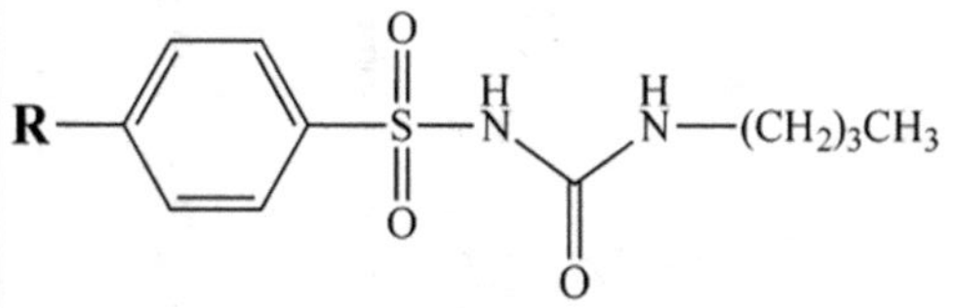

R	Human plasma $t_{1/2}$
CH_3 (tolbutamide)	5.9 h
Cl (chlorpropamide)	33 h

Celecoxib is metabolized by CYP2C9 on the benzylic methyl position. In rat, modification of CH_3 to CF_3 lowers the clearance and hence longer plasma half life (Ahlström et al. 2007).
Target: COX-2 inhibitor

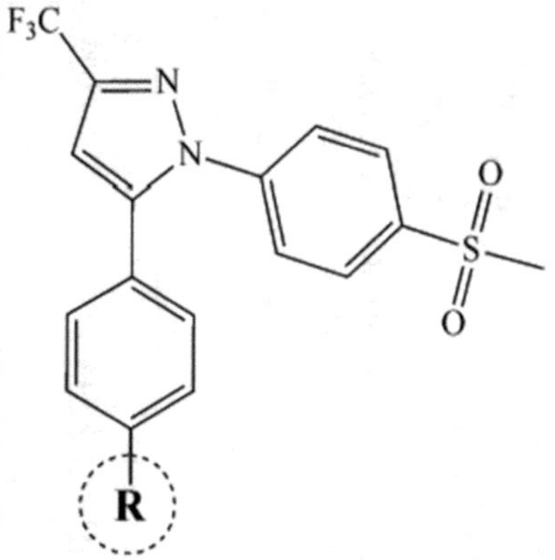

	R	$t_{1/2}$ (h)
Celecoxib	CH_3	3.5
	CF_3	220

Three sites of metabolism (**A-C**) were modified (Rohde et al. 2007).

1. A prevented a lipophilic site oxidation.
2. B blocked by methyl
3. C blocked by CF3
Target: 11β-hydroxysteroid dehydrogenase-1

CLint (L/h/kg)
Mouse 380 → 7
Human 110 → 3

Case 3.5: Using 1-aminobenzotriazole (ABT) in drug discovery

1-Aminobenzotriazole (ABT) is a non-selective mechanism-based inactivator of CYP isoforms except for CYP2C9 (de Montellano 2018). It is used both in vitro and in vivo for silencing the CYP metabolic clearance in relatively high concentrations (mM). Relatively selective except for inhibiting N-acetyl transferases (NAT) that ABT is the substrate of.

For CYP2C9 inhibition, addition of (S)-warfarin, resulted in switching ABT from poor to potent inactivator of this enzyme (Sodhi et al. 2014).

Toxicity: No overt toxicity is observed when administering ABT to animals. This is consistent with 16-day study in mouse (Watanabe et al. 2016) and 13-week study in rats (Meschter et al. 1994). In rat hepatic CYP levels and resorufin dealkylation activity were reduced to less than 30% of control values without obvious signs of toxicity such as changes in body weight, food consumption, or clinical appearance.

Experimental procedures:

In vitro, ABT (1 mM) requires at least 15 min of pre-incubation in the presence of the enzyme and NADPH.

In vivo, ABT inactivates CYP isoforms at po doses of 50 mg/kg in rats, and 20 mg/kg in dogs and monkeys. Under these conditions, the plasma concentrations are high and are sustained for over 24 h (Balani et al. 2002). Mike Fisher et al. argued that ABT given orally or iv could elucidate factors limiting oral bioavailability (Strelevitz et al. 2006). In rats, there is an observation of delayed gastric emptying time (Stringer et al. 2014).

1-Aminobenzotriazole ⟶ [P450] ⟶ (benzyne intermediate) ⟶ Benzyne + $2N_2$ ⟶ Covalent binding to P450 resulting in its inactivation

3.4.1.2 Aldehyde Oxidase (AO)

Subcellular location: Cytosol.

Organ distribution: Highest levels in the liver, followed by the lung, kidney and small intestine.

Isoforms: Humans have one AO, rodents have 4 and dogs have none. Female rodents generally have greater AO functional activity than do male rodents. The active site of AOs in humans is the largest among the species and, therefore, accommodates more diverse substrates.

Several drugs have failed in the market due to the involvement of AO metabolism. The challenge observed in few cases were the increase clearance or toxicity. The clearance in many examples were not predicted by the preclinical species tested plus the in vitro system was lacking the right tissue fraction. Fortunately, the use of hepatocytes has alleviated the absence of some of the hepatic enzymes in fractions such as liver microsomes.

Computational approaches: By combing electronic and steric factors for heteroaromatic moieties (Xu et al. 2017; Jones and Korzekwa 2013) (Fig. 3.9).

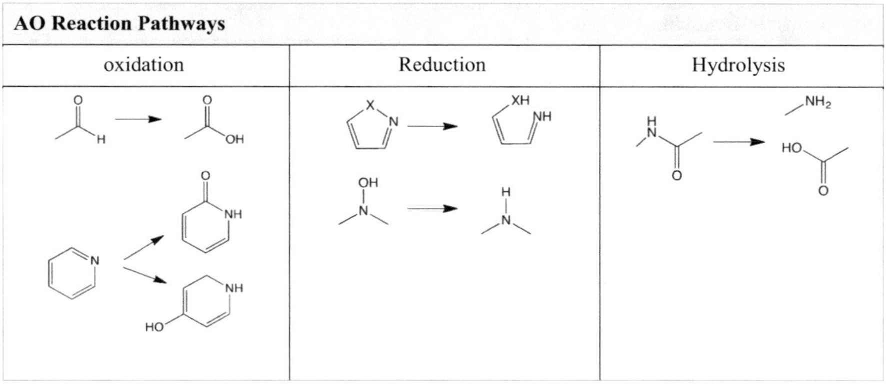

AO Reaction Pathways

oxidation	Reduction	Hydrolysis

Fig. 3.9 Typical aldehyde oxidase (AO) reaction pathways

Case 3.6: Novel AO Role in Hydrolysis

A clinical candidate, GDC-0834 (BTK inhibitor), failed in the due to high clearance. This was shown based on hepatocytes in human but at the time of progressing the molecule to the clinic.

Further studies were conducted: (1) tissue fractionation, (2) enzymatic activity, (3) proteomics, followed (4) chemical inhibitors This calls out aldehyde oxidase (AO) as the enzyme responsbile for the hydrolytic reaction of GDC-0834. This was confirmed with using AO substrates and inhibitors (Sodhi et al. 2015).

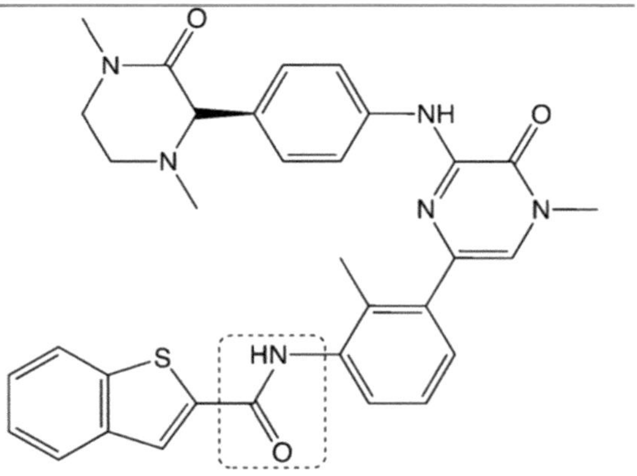

GDC-0834

Strategies to Removing AO Liability

Strategies to remove AO involvement	
Decrease Risk factor Increase nitrogen count on the ring 5-membered ring size e-donating Manevski et al. 2019	

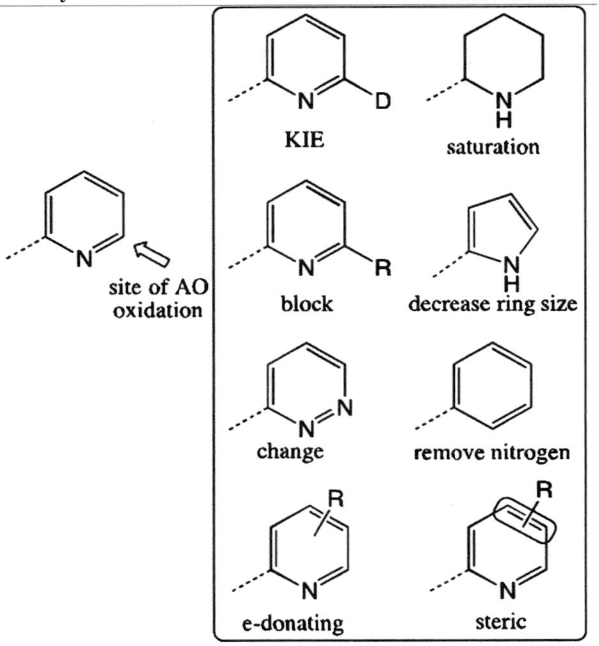

Case 3.7: AO Contribution to (1) High Clearance, (2) Low Bioavailability, and (3) Renal Toxicity

High Clearance RO1 has a short half (0.7 h) in human but the predicted to be much higher (~6 h) (El-Kattan and Varma 2018; Zhang et al. 2011) 1. AO contributed to significant oxidative metabolite that was further glucuronidated together account for >700% of the *AUC* of the parent. 2. The metabolites were minor in preclinical species (rat, dog, monkey).	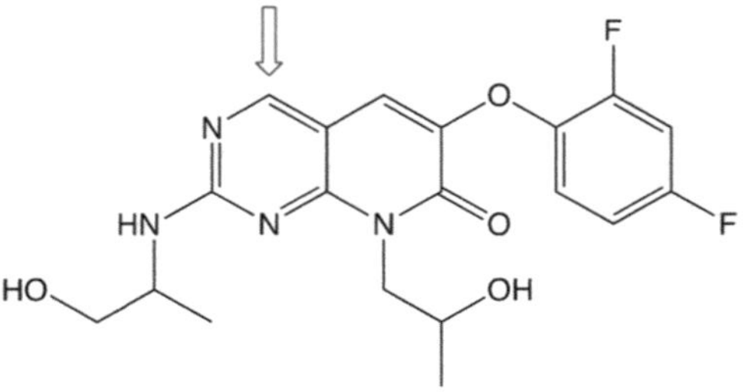 RO1 Arrow: site of AO oxidation
Low bioavailability **FK3453** has low oral bioavailability in human. Liver microsomes also reported low turn-over (expected from a cytosolic enzymes). Rat and dog were not good models for predicting AO metabolism in human (Akabane et al. 2011). Target: Adenosine A1/2 dual inhibitor for Parkinson's disease.	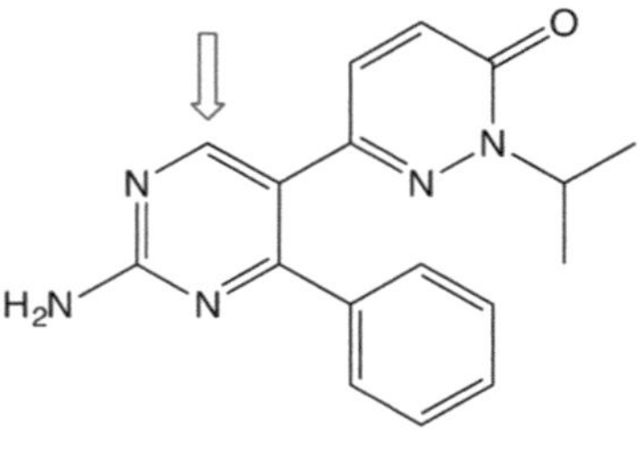 FK3453 Arrow: Site of AO oxidation

Renal toxicity **SGX523** and **JNJ-38877605:** Caused kidney toxicity in patients treated. This was due to poor solubility of the AO-mediated metabolites (Diamond et al. 2010; Lolkema et al. 2015). 1. The metabolite in each case crystalized in renal tubulin that eventually lead to renal toxicity. 2. The AO metabolite was not formed significantly in rat, and dog. **Target:** c-met tyrosine kinase inhibitor	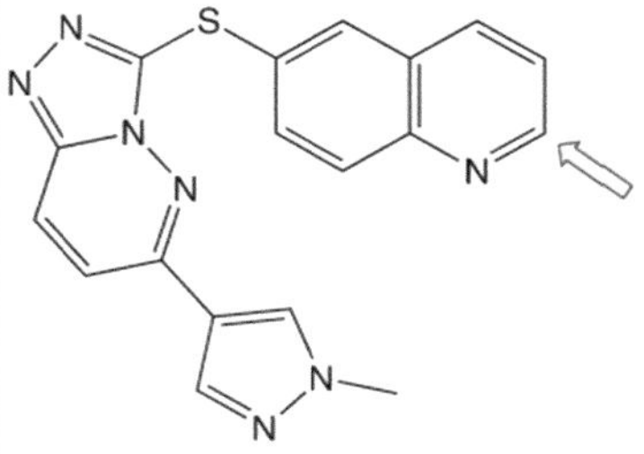 SGX523 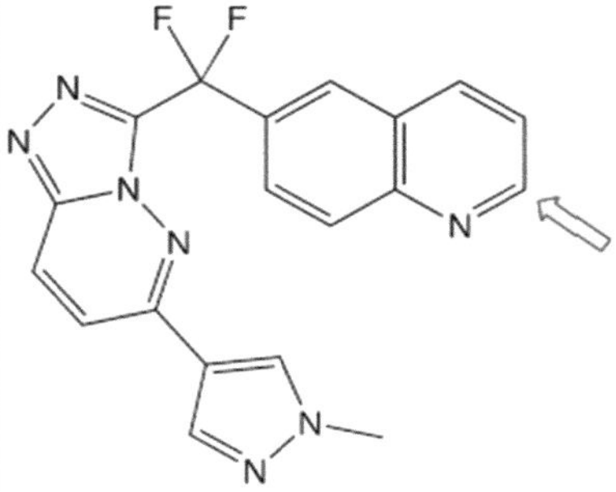 JNJ-38877605

3.4.1.3   Flavin Containing Monooxygenase (FMO)

FMO oxidizes secondary/tertiary amines (pKa range 8–11) to generate *N*-oxidation product (Cruciani et al. 2014). Primary amines are weak substrates of FMO. Same reaction could be performed by CYP so knowing differences between enzymes are important.

FMO vs CYP: (1) FMO is inactivated by heating at 45 °C for 10 min minus NADPH, (2) SKF-525A is a potent inhibitor of FMO and not CYP.

In adult human

FMO-1	kidney > > lung, small intestine > > liver
FMO-2	lung > > kidney > liver, small intestine
FMO-3 (major)	liver > > lung > kidney > > small intestine
FMO-4	liver > kidney > lung > small intestine
FMO-5	liver > > small intestine, lung, kidney

FMO-3 preclinical species

Liver:	rabbit > rat, humans > dog > mouse
Kidney:	rat > rabbit > mouse > dog

Sex Differences:	females of mouse and dog have higher activity than males
FMO Inhibitors:	methimazole and thiourea
Enhancers of FMO:	N-octylamine

Case 3.8: FMO Substrates

FMO3 metabolizes a limited range of substrates compared to CYPs. For example, although below four compounds are very similar from a three-dimensional point of view, they showed different specificity to FMO3. **1** and **2** are FMO3 substrates while **3** and **4** are not).

Crystalline structures of yeast and bacterial isoforms of FMO have been reported which provide a reasonable base for the human FMO (Cruciani et al. 2014).

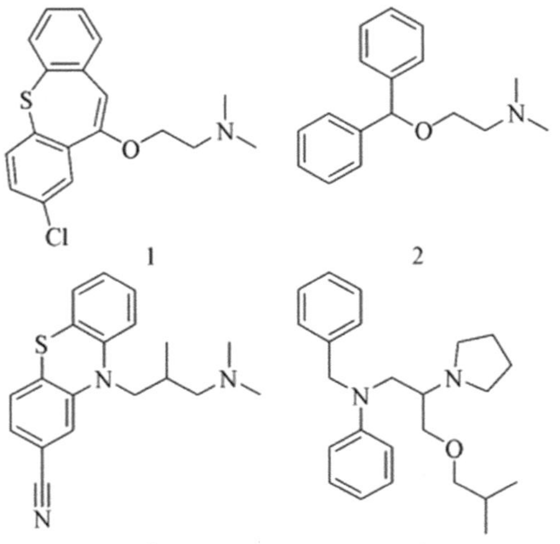

3.4.1.4   Epoxide Hydrolase (EH)

Reactions: Hydrolysis of arene and alkene epoxides to polar diols.

The two classes of EH that are important for xenobiotic metabolism are microsomal EH (mEH; prefers *cis* epoxide substrates; optimum pH = 9) and soluble EH (sEH; prefers *trans* epoxide substrates; optimum pH = 7.4). (Morisseau and Hammock 2005).

Organ distribution: Both types are present in all tissues, with the highest level in the liver.

The hydrolysis of epoxides plays a key role in detoxification (for example, the hydrolysis of epoxide derivatives of polycyclic aromatic hydrocarbons such as benzo[a]pyrene 4,5-oxide).

mEH substrates: Benzo[a]pyrene 4,5-oxide, cis-stilbene oxide and styrene oxide.

mEH inhibitors: 1,1,1-Trichloropropene-2,3-oxide, divalent heavy metals (Hg^{2+} and Zn^{2+}) and cyclopropyl oxiranes.

sEH substrate: *Trans*-stilbene oxide.

sEH inhibitors: Chalcone oxides, *trans*-3-phenylglycidols, Cd^{2+} and Cu^{2+}.

Case 3.9: Blocking mEH Metabolism

Oxetane SAR of hydrolysis by human mEH (Toselli et al. 2017).
1. Methyl spacer (i.e., n = 1) increased the oxetane hydrolysis.
2. Substitution on R_1 or R_2 alone did not significantly affect hydrolysis.
3. Combination of substitution and introduction of spacer greatly improve hydrolysis.

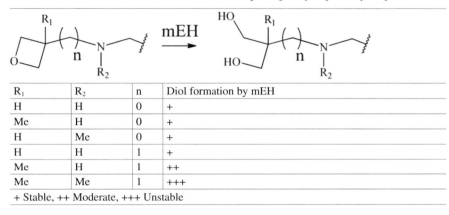

R_1	R_2	n	Diol formation by mEH
H	H	0	+
Me	H	0	+
H	Me	0	+
H	H	1	+
Me	H	1	++
Me	Me	1	+++

+ Stable, ++ Moderate, +++ Unstable

3.4.1.5 Uridine Diphosphate Glucuronosyltransferases (UGT)

Localized on the luminal side of the ER and are present liver, kidney and intestine. Cofactor: Uridine diphosphoglucuronic acid (UDPGA).

- Typically, the glucuronides are considered to be the final metabolic products. However, other metabolic modifications have been reported, including diglucuronide conjugates. Gemifibrozil glucuronide is a potent inhibitor of CYP2C8 (Ogilvie et al. 2006).
- A number of transporters (mostly hepatic such as MRP3 and MRP2) are known to transport glucuronide conjugates.
- Sometimes, albeit rarely, glucuronides have significant pharmacological activity (i.e., morphine glucuronide).
- Quantification of the parent drug is conducted in the presence and absence of β-glucuronidase to regenerate the aglycan parent. The difference in quantification will be the amount of glucuronide metabolite formed.

> **Considerations for In Vitro Incubations:**
> Detergents (Brij 58, lubrol and triton X-100) or alamethicin provide access to the luminal side of the ER.
>
> - Alamethicin is a pore-forming peptide; it should be dissolved in methanol and mixed with microsomes (20–50 µg/mg LM) on ice for 15–20 min prior to incubation.
> - Detergents inhibit CYP activity, and since a number of metabolites are formed by CYP and UGT enzymes, alamethicin is used more often than detergents in *in vitro* incubations.
>
> 1,4-Saccharolactone inhibits β-glucuronidase activity.

Acyl Glucuronides

A number of glucuronide conjugates of carboxylic acids (acyl glucuronides) are considered reactive electrophilic metabolites. They are capable of undergoing hydrolysis, intramolecular rearrangement, and intermolecular reactions with proteins leading to covalent drug/protein adducts. A number of acyl glucuronides lead to idiosyncratic hepatotoxicity that is considered to be immune mediated.

Glucuronide Chemical Stability

Glucuronides of primary and secondary amines are acid labile.
    Acyl glucuronides are base labile (Table 3.9).

Case 3.11: Species Differences in N-Glucuronidation Formation

A (mTOR inhibitor) undergoes extensive *N*-glucuronidation (sites **1–3**) (Berry et al. 2014).

Species differences:

1. Sites **1–3** glucuronide metabolites formed in liver of rat, dog, and human, while site **3** not detected in cynomolgus monkey.
2. Higher rates of clearance due to N-glucuronidation for monkey and human.
3. Monkeys may not be a good animal model for human *N*-glucuronidation by UGT1A9 or UGT1A1.

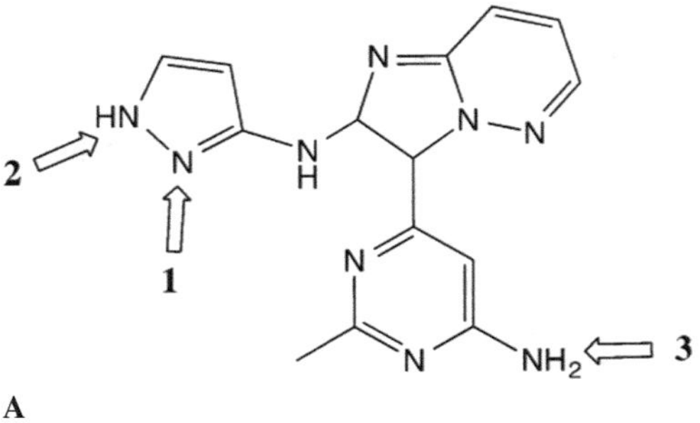

Table 3.9 Major sites of UGT expression and the enzymes' substrates and inhibitors

UGT[a]	Tissue	Substrates	Inhibitors
1A1 (15%)	Liver, intestine	Bilirubin, β-estradiol, ethynylestradiol, morphine, SN-38	Atazanavir
1A3	Liver	Bile acids, cyproheptadine, alizarin, hyodeoxycholic acid	
1A4 (20%)	Liver	Imipramine, trifluoroperazine	Hecogenin
1A5	Liver, brain		
1A6	Liver, brain	Seratonin, naphthol	Amitriptyline, phenylbutazone
1A7	Stomach		Phenylbutazone, sulfinpyrizone
1A8	Intestine		
1A9	Liver, kidney	Propofol	Androsterone, phenylbutazone, sulfinpyrizone
1A10	Stomach, intestine		Amitriptyline
2B4	Liver	Xenobiotics, bile acids, hyodeoxycholic acid	
2B7 (35%)	Liver, kidney, intestine	AZT, morphine	Amitriptyline, androsterone
2B10	Liver, prostate, mammary		
2B11	Liver, kidney, prostate, adrenal		
2B15	Liver, prostate	(S)-Oxazepam	Amitriptyline, quinidine, quinine
2B17	Prostate		Amitriptyline, quinidine, quinine

Uchaipichat et al. (2006)
[a]Percent of marketed drugs that are metabolized by the major UGT enzymes (Williams et al. 2004)
AZT 3′-azido-3′-deoxythimidine

3.4.2   Optimization Based on Metabolism of Isosteres

During drug discovery, molecules are being synthesized for optimized different properties with one being for metabolic stability. Initially as molecules are being assessed in in vitro metabolic stability such as hepatocytes, the factors involved may not know the drug metabolizing enzymes or the type of metabolites formed. For these reasons it is important to have familiarities on the type of moieties and reactions. Here we summarize examples for this purpose.

Case 3.12: Isosteres for Optimizing Hydrolytic Reactions

Stability from esters, amides, carbamates, and urea (Ghosh and Brindisi 2019)

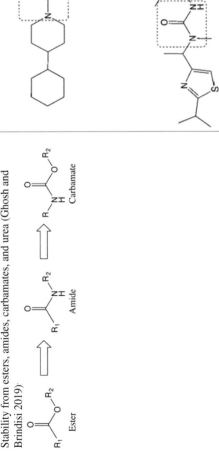

Ritonavir

Ritonavir was discovered by optimizing metabolic hot spots at the tail end of a linear peptidomimetic molecule (in A-80987).
Site **A**: Replacing two terminal pyridines that were metabolic oxidative hot spots by two thiazole.
Site **B**: replacing a carbamate with a more soluble *N*-methylurea resulted in increased the oral bioavailability from 0% to 78% (Kempf et al. 1998).

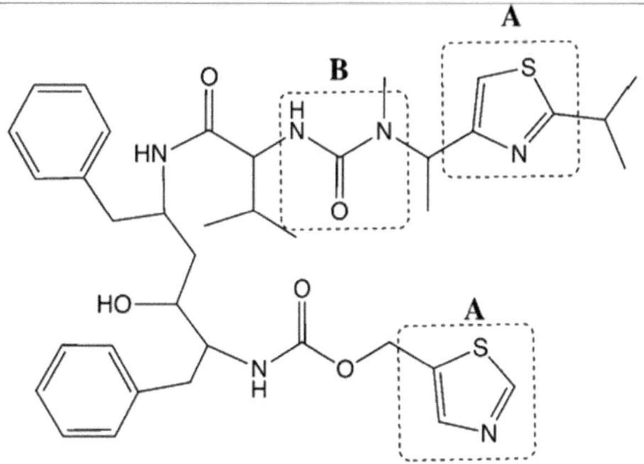

Ritonavir

Procaine local anesthetic with very short duration of action due to rapid hydrolysis by esterases.
Lidocaine has longer duration due to better stability gained by:
1. Changes to amide plus steric block to prevent hydrolysisDimethyl ortho to the amide for blocking hydrolysis

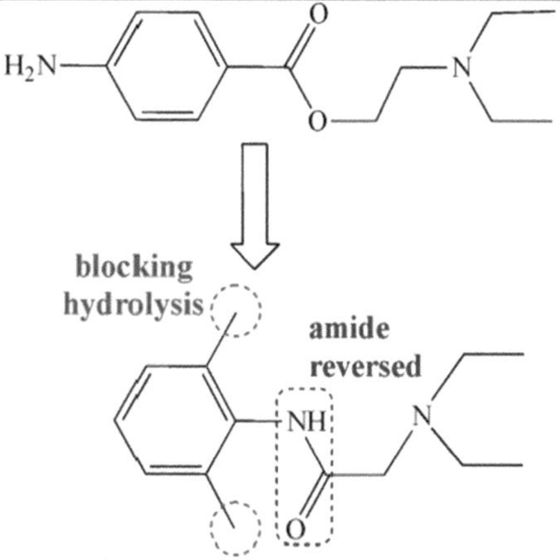

Case 3.12: Isosters of Replacing Phenyl with Fluoro-pyrazole for Blood Stability

A was metabolically unstable in blood. Replacement of phenyl ring with 4-fluoropyrazole (**B**) improved the stability in the blood (Pei et al. 2018).
Target: TDO2 inhibitor

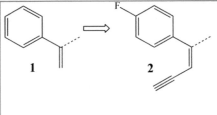

A   **B**

Case 3.13: Changes that Resulted in Metabolic Stability

Enviradene (1) Was Metabolically Unstable. With Two Modifications, The Molecule Was Both Active And Metabolically Stable (Victor et al. 1997).
The Changes Were:
1. Para-Fluoro Substitution
2. *Trans*-Vinylacetylene (May Increase Bioactivation Potential?)
Target: Rhinovirus Induced "Common Cold"

Case 3.14: Molecular Matched Pair for Optimization of Metabolic Rates

Matched molecular pair analysis is a powerful mechnaism to learn from existing dataset.
A series of cycloalkyl ether were examined (Stepan et al. 2012) and here are few take-home messages:
1. reduction of ring size THP to THF to Oxetane
2. change of *O*-substitution position on the ring decrease CL_{int} 2-substitued to 3- or 4-substituted

Transformation	$CL_{int,u}$*
2-THP → 2-THF	−13.4
2-THF → 2-oxetane	−31.4
3-THP → 3-THF	−22.7
3-THF → 3-oxetane	−18.3
2-THP → 2-oxetane	−65.4
3-THP → 3-oxetane	−45.1
2-THP → 3-THP	−19.8
2-THP → 4-THP	−17.6
3-THP → 4-THP	−23.8
2-THF → 3-THF	−4.5
2-oxetane → 3-oxetane	−25.4

In human liver microsomes in mL/min/kg

Case 3.15: Isosteres of Morpholine with Lowering Clearance

There is a large number of nitrogen-containing aliphatic rings used in drug design (Kumari and Singh 2020). They include: morpholine, piperazine, piperidine, pyrrolidine, aziridine, azetidine, and azepane

Drug metabolizing enzymes: Typically involves CYP plus at times MAO, AO and Phase II enzymes (Bolleddula et al. 2014). The common reactions are *N*-oxidation, oxidative *N*-dealkylation, ring oxidation and *N*-conjugation.

Metabolic fate of morpholine.

Morpholine metabolism is mainly oxidative by nature that could result in secondary and tertiary metabolites. The phase 2 conjugation reactions except for methylation are not captured here.

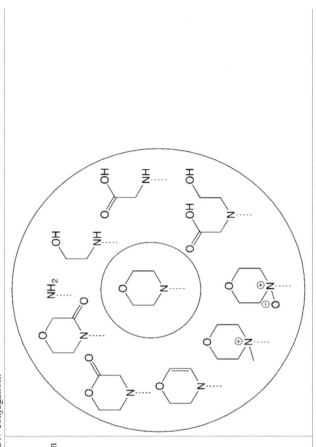

TPSA 83110
logP 2.8 1.1

Entospletinib is extensively matabolized on the morpholino ring. Modification of morpholine to *N*-oxatane piperizine resulted eventually the discovery of lanraplenib.[137] This also translated into less frequent dosing for lanraplenib from twice daily to once daily. **Target:** Spleen tyrosine kinase (SYK) inhibitor for signaling in a variety of immune cell types such as B-cells, monocytes, and macrophages to treat autoimmune and inflammatory diseases.

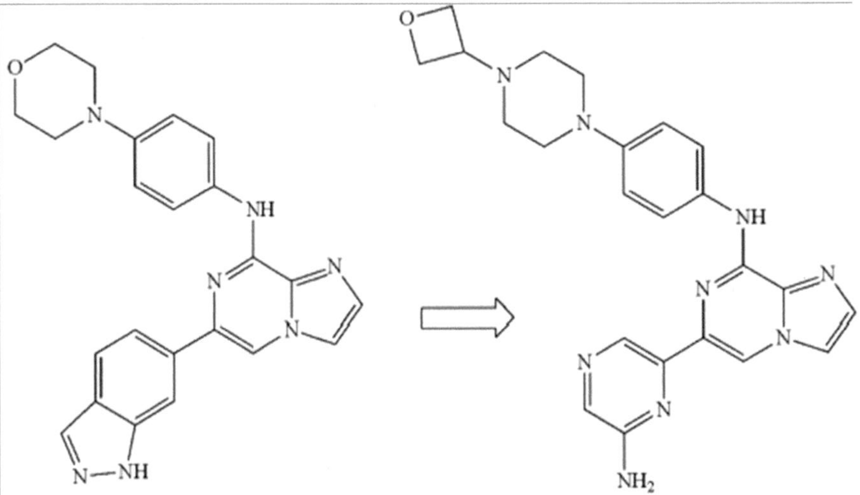

Metabolic fate of Piperazine

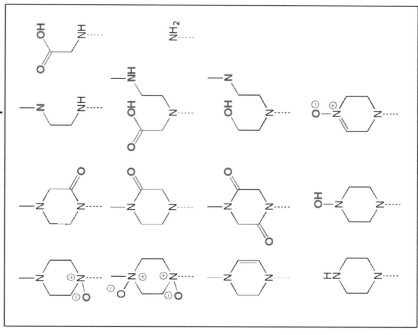

Case 3.16: Isosters of Phenyl to Pyridine to Improve Solubility and Metabolic Stability

A has poor solubility and metabolic stability and making **B** (phenyl to pyridine by incorporation of a nitrogen atom) significantly improve these properties (Siegrist et al. 2016).

Target: T-type calcium channels.

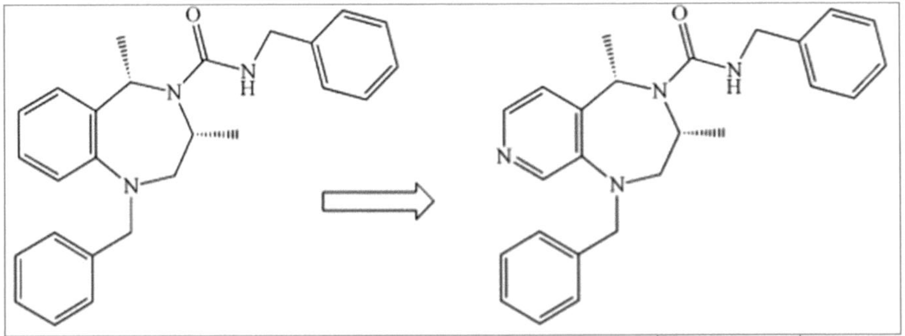

A		
		B
Properties	A	B
Solubility (µg/mL, pH - 7)	<1	27
HLM CL_{int} (µL/min/mg protein)	>1250	56
TPSA	36	61
logP	4.1	3.0

Case 3.17: Type I And II Binding of Pyridine to CYP Resulting in Inhibition

CYP substrate have two different types of binding:

Type I. results in high-spin iron (III)

Type II. the molecule binds to heme-iron and results in low-spin iron (III)

SAR of binding for a series of Quinoline Carboxamide Analogues by CYP3A4 (Dahal et al. 2011).

R_2= N(CH$_3$)$_2$, OCH$_3$, H, CH$_3$,

R_1=

| Series | 1 | 2 | 3 | 4 | 5 |

Type I: N-demethylation > O-demethylation ~ benzylic hydroxylation > aromatic hydroxylation.

Type II: N-demethylation> bezylic hydroxylation > O-demethylation ~aromatic hydroxylation

Case 3.18: Fluoro Substitution Resulted in Removal of CYP3A4 Time-Dependent Inhibitor

1 is a CYP3A4 a TDI.

Difluoro substitution (**2**) eliminated the TDI of CYP3A4 (Wu et al. 2003). This is thought to be through blocking formation of quinone-type intermediate on each of the rings by CYP3A4.

	R1	R2	TDI
1	H	H	Yes
2	F	F	No

3.5 Permeability and Drug Transporters

This chapter supplies basic information about the assessment of drug permeability across biological membranes and drug transporters. Drug permeability is often assessed using *in vitro* assays, some of which are described in Chap. 6. Transporters are membrane proteins that play a role in the movement of endogenous substances and xenobiotics across cellular membranes into and out of cells and are evaluated largely by *in vitro* assays.

3.5.1 Basic Concepts and Definitions

Apical
The apical or luminal membrane is the surface of the membrane that faces the lumen.

Basolateral
The basolateral membrane is the surface of the membrane that forms the basal and lateral surfaces and faces away from the lumen (blood side).

Canalicular
The canalicular membrane is the surface of a hepatocyte membrane that is facing the bile duct. The canicular membrane is the apical membrane of a hepatocyte.

Sinusoidal
The sinusoidal membrane is the surface of a hepatocyte membrane facing the sinusoids and is the basolateral membrane of a hepatocyte.

Influx and Efflux Transporters
Influx transporters are those that move substrates into cells whereas efflux transporters are those that pump substrates out of cells. Examples include P-glycoprotein (P-gp, MDR1, ABCB1) which is perhaps the best-known efflux transporter and organic anion transporting polypeptides (OATPs) which are examples of influx transporters.

Absorptive and Secretory Transporters
Absorptive transporters are transporters that transfer substrates into the systemic blood circulation. In contrast, secretory transporters are those that transfer substrates out of the systemic blood circulation into the gut lumen, bile or urine.

ATP-binding cassette (ABC) transporters and solute carrier (SLC) transporters are the two main classes that drug transporters can be categorized into.

ABC Transporters
The ABC family of transporters requires ATP hydrolysis in order to transport substrates across membranes. Therefore, ABC transporters are primarily active transporters. Notable examples of ABC transporters include P-gp, multidrug resistance-associated protein (MRP) and breast cancer resistance protein (BCRP). The following are brief descriptions of select ABC transporters:

P-glycoprotein (P-gp, MDR1, ABCB1) P-gp is involved in the ATP-dependent efflux of xenobiotics from cells and is probably the best characterized of all transporters. It was discovered originally as a result of its ability to confer resistance of tumors to anti-cancer drugs. P-gp is found to be expressed in the intestine, kidney, liver and the brain. It plays a role in limiting the entry of certain drugs through the blood-brain barrier. It can also play a role in intestinal absorption and in biliary and urinary excretion. Digoxin is the best characterized of the P-gp substrates.

Breast Cancer Resistance Protein (BCRP, MXR) BCRP is a half ABC transporter that is expressed in the gastrointestinal tract (intestine and colon), liver, kidney, brain, mammary tissues, testes, and the placenta. Similar to P-gp, BCRP was initially discovered due to its ability to confer resistance to cancer cell lines in vitro. BCRP plays a role in limiting oral bioavailability of certain drugs and limits entry of selected substrates through the blood-brain barrier, blood-testis barrier and the blood-placenta barrier.

SLC Transporters

In contrast to ABC transporters, SLC transporters do not have ATP-binding sites. Transport by SLC transporters use either an electrochemical potential difference in the substrate (i.e. facilitated transporters) or an ion gradient across membranes produced by primary active transporters and transport substrates against an electrochemical difference (i.e. secondary active transporters). Examples of SLC transporters include OATPs, organic anion transporters (OAT), organic cation transporters (OCT), etc. Most known drug uptake transporters are SLC transporters. The following are brief descriptions of select SLC transports:

Organic Cation Transporter (OCT) and Organic anion Transporter (OAT) OCTs and OATs are found in kidney and play a role in the excretion of cations and anions (xenobiotics or endogenous), respectively, into the urine. They can also be found in other tissues such as hepatocytes where they act primarily as uptake transporters and intestinal epithelia (OCT1).

Organic Anion Transporting Polypeptides (OATP) OATPs are involved in the sodium-independent transport of a diverse range of amphiphilic organic compounds including bile acids, thyroid hormones and steroid conjugates and many xenobiotics. OATPs can be found in liver, intestine, kidney and blood-brain barrier. This transporter appears to be involved in clinically relevant transporter drug-drug interactions that are of the largest magnitude.

Multidrug and toxin extrusion (MATE) proteins MATE proteins are transporters of metabolic and xenobiotic organic cations. They are expressed in the liver on the canalicular membrane (apical) of hepatocytes, and the kidney on the brush-border membrane (apical, urine side) of proximal tubule cells. MATE1 shows high expression in skeletal muscle cells.

Human and Rodent Nomenclature

In general, human genes and proteins are designated in capitals. Rodent genes and proteins are designated with a capital letter followed by lower case letters. For example, SLCO and OATP are the human gene and protein for organic anion transporting polypeptides. The analogous rodent gene and protein for organic anion transporting polypeptides are designated as Slco and Oatp, respectively.

Permeability and Efflux Ratio

Permeability is the measure of the ability of a drug to cross passively cross biological membranes. Permeability as a property provides insight on whether a xenobiotic can cross the intestinal membrane and potentially have good oral bioavailability. For xenobiotics that are designed to act on a specific tissue (i.e. brain for CNS drugs), permeability provides insight on the ability to enter these targets and elicit the desired biological effect.

Permeability is determined commonly using cell culture-based models utilizing Caco-2 cells (a continuous line of heterogeneous human epithelial colorectal adenocarcinoma cells) or MDCK cells (Madin-Darby Canine Kidney Cells). In studies where the contribution of specific transporters is examined, MDCK cells overexpressing a particular transporter of interest are often utilized. Examples of such MDCK cell lines include MDR1-MDCK (P-gp over-expressing cells) and MRP2-MDCK II cells (MRP2 over-expressing cells).

In brief, cells are grown on permeable culture inserts in transwells until they reach full confluence. Compound is applied to either the apical or basolateral side of the cell monolayer depending on whether permeability is being measured from apical to basolateral or vice versa. Permeability is determined as follows:

$$P_{app} = \frac{dR}{dt} \times \frac{1}{AC_{Donar\_initial}} \tag{3.14}$$

where P_{app} is the apparent permeability

dR/dt is the rate of appearance of the compound in the receiver side (i.e. if compound is applied to the apical side, the basolateral side is the receiver).
A is area of the transwell insert.
$C_{Donar\_initial}$ is the initial concentration on the donor side at time 0.

In established cellular assays assessing permeability (MDCK and Caco-2), Table 3.10 provides how compounds are categorized as low, moderate and high permeability. It must be noted that established assays should contain appropriate positive controls of known permeability.

Table 3.10 Cell-based permeability categories

Cellular assay	P_{app} (AB) ($\times 10^{-6}$ cm/sec)		
	Low	Moderate	High
MDCK and Caco-2	< 1	1–10	> 10

$^a P_{app}$ (AB) is the apparent permeability from the apical to basolateral side in an *in vitro* permeability assay

For investigations of transporters, an efflux ratio is determined using the appropriate in vitro cellular assay. The efflux ratio (*ER*) is determined using an in vitro system and is defined as:

$$ER = \frac{P_{app}(BA)}{P_{app}(AB)} \tag{3.15}$$

where

P_{app} *(BA)* is the apparent permeability from the basolateral to apical side in an *in vitro* permeability assay.

P_{app} *(AB)* is the apparent permeability from the apical to basolateral side in an *in vitro* permeability assay.

P_{app} (BA) > P_{app} (AB) suggests an efflux ratio (of >1). Practically speaking, ER ≥ 2 is suggestive of the presence of efflux. Efflux ratios can also vary with the cellular system used. For example, a compound can have an efflux ratio of approximately 1 in an assay using Caco-2 cells but can have an efflux ratio > 3 in a MDR1-MDCK assay. In this case, the higher efflux ratio observed in MDR1-MDCK cells may be related to the degree of over-expression of MDR1 (P-gp) in the MDR1-MDCK cells.

The incorporation of the impact of transporters into physiologically based pharmacokinetic models is still in its infancy. Although the necessary theory is available, insufficient information is available on the expression of transporters in various tissues and their maximum capacity to transport various substrates in humans.

3.5.2   Localization of Select Transporters

The blood-brain barrier is unique in that the basolateral membrane of brain capillary endothelial cells faces the brain rather than the blood. In the intestine, liver and kidney, the basolateral membrane faces the blood.

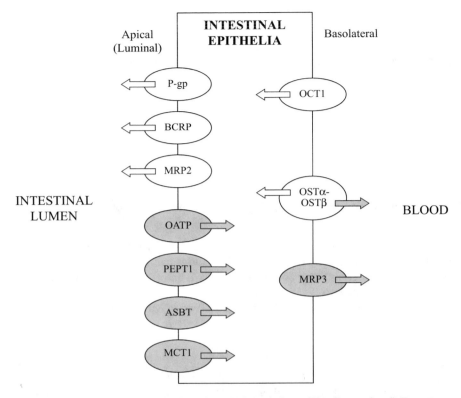

Fig. 3.10 Select transporters in intestine. (Adapted from The International Transporter Consortium 2010)

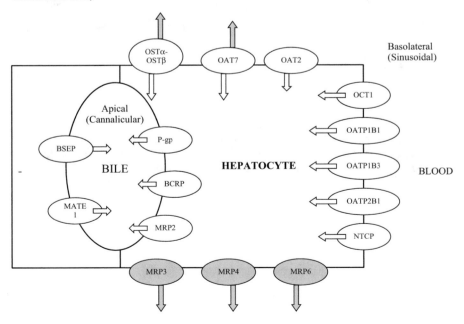

Fig. 3.11 Select transporters in liver. (Adapted from The International Transporter Consortium 2010)

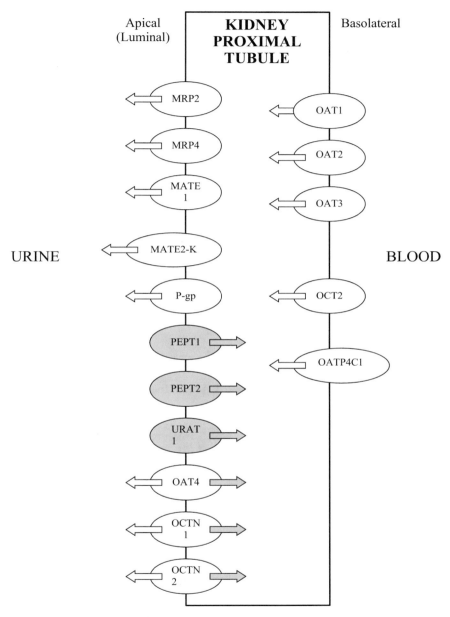

Fig. 3.12 Select transporters in kidney. (Adapted from The International Transporter Consortium 2010)

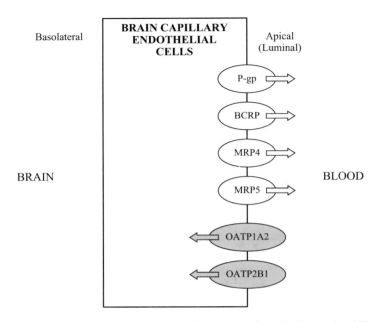

Fig. 3.13 Select transporters at blood-brain barrier. (Adapted from The International Transporter Consortium 2010).

Table 3.11 Localization of select ABC transporters. Adapted from The International Transporter Consortium 2010

Transporter (Alias)	Gene	Location (Organs/Cells)
MDR1 (P-gp, ABCB1)	*ABCB1*	Intestinal enterocytes, kidney proximal tubule, hepatocytes (canalicular), brain endothelia
MDR3 (ABCB4)	*ABCB4*	Hepatocytes (canalicular)
BCRP (MXR)	*ABCG2*	Intestinal enterocytes, hepatocytes (canalicular), kidney proximal tubule, brain endothelia, placenta, stem cells, mammary glands (lactating)
MRP2 (ABCC2, cMOAT)	*ABCC2*	Hepatocytes (canalicular), kidney (proximal tubule, luminal), enterocytes (luminal)
MRP3 (ABCC3)	*ABCC3*	Hepatocytes (sinusoidal), intestinal enterocytes (basolateral)
MRP4 (ABCC4)	*ABCC4*	Kidney proximal tubule (luminal), choroid plexus, hepatocytes (sinusoidal), platelets
BSEP (SPGP, cBAT, ABCB11)	*ABCB11*	Hepatocytes canalicular

Table 3.12 Localization of select SLC transporters

Transporter (Alias)	Gene	Location (Organs/Cells)
OATP1A2 (OATP-A)	*SLCO1A2*	Brain capillaries endothelia, cholangiocytes, distal nephron
OATP1B1 (OATP-C, OATP2, LST-1)	*SLCO1B1*	Hepatocytes (sinusoidal)
OATP1B3 (OATP-8)	*SLCO1B3*	Hepatocytes (sinusoidal)
OATP2B1 (OATP-B)	*SLCO2B1*	Hepatocytes (sinusoidal), endothelia
OAT1	*SLC22A6*	Kidney proximal tubule, placenta
OAT3	*SLC22A8*	Kidney proximal tubule, choroid plexus, blood-brain barrier
OCT1	*SLC22A1*	Hepatocytes (sinusoidal), intestinal enterocytes
OCT2	*SLC22A2*	Kidney proximal tubule, neurons
PEPT1	SLC15A1	Intestinal enterocytes, kidney proximal tubule
PEPT2	SLC15A2	Kidney proximal tubule, choroid plexus, lung
MATE1	SLC47A1	Kidney proximal tubule, liver (canalicular membrane), skeletal muscle
MATE2-K	SLC47A2	Kidney proximal tubule

Adapted from The International Transporter Consortium (2010)

3.5.3 Transporters of Interest for Evaluation

Currently, investigational drugs are suggested to be evaluated as substrates or inhibitors of the following transporters based on interaction with compounds that are in clinically in use.

- P-gp
- BCRP
- OATP1B1/ OATP1B3
- OAT1/ OAT3
- OCT2
- MATE1/MATE2-K

The timing of the evaluation during the drug discovery phase is highly dependent on the need-to-know information about transporters for a specific series of compounds as many of the assays used determine a compound's transporter substrate/inhibition characteristics are not as routinely employed early on in drug discovery. An example of a situation where transporter information may be gathered earlier is for neuroscience programs especially if a chemical series being optimized suffers from being P-gp substrates. Finally, unlike the situation for CYP enzymes, specific *in vitro* methods to determine induction of transporters is not well established.

Substrates and Inhibitors
Substrates and inhibitors of transporters are, in general, less selective than substrates and inhibitors of CYP enzymes (Table 3.13). The following are tables summarizing known substrates and inhibitors of select ABC and SLC transporters. It should be noted that many of substrates and inhibitors listed are not selective for specific transporters (Table 3.14).

Table 3.13 Select examples of *in vitro* transporter substrates and inhibitors

Transporter	Substrate	Inhibitor
P-gp	Digoxin, fexofenadine, loperamide, quinidine, talinolol, vinblastine	Cyclosporine, elacridar (GF120918), ketoconazole, quinidine, reserpine, ritonavir, tacrolimus, valspodar (PSC833), verapamil, zosuquidar (LY335979)
BCRP	2-amino-1-methyl-6-phenylimidazo[4,5-β]pyridine (PhIP), coumestrol, daidzein, dantrolene, estrone-3-sulfate, genistein, prazosin, sulfasalazine	Elacridar (GF120918), fumitremorgin C, Ko134, Ko143, novobiocin, sulfasalazine
OATP1B1, OATP1B3	Cholecystokinin octapeptide (CCK-8), estradiol-17β-glucuronide, estrone-3-sulfate, pitavastatin, pravastatin, telmisartan, rosuvastatin	Cyclosporine, estradiol-17β-glucuronide, estrone-3-sulfate, rifampicin, rifamycin SV
OAT1	Adefovir, *p*-aminohippurate, cidofovir, tenofovir	Benzylpenicillin, probenecid
OAT3	Benzylpenicillin, estrone-3-sulfate, methotrexate, pravastatin	
MATE1, MATE-2 K	Metformin, 1-methyl-4-phenylpyridinium (MPP+), tetraethylammonium (TEA)	Cimetidine, pyrimethamine
OCT2	Metformin, 1-methyl-4-phenylpyridinium (MPP+), tetraethylammonium (TEA)	Cimetidine

https://www.fda.gov/drugs/drug-interactions-labeling/drug-development-and-drug-interactions-table-substrates-inhibitors-and-inducers(Accessed on 5-10-2021)

Table 3.14 Select examples of *in vivo* clinical transporter substrates and inhibitors

Transporter	Substrate	Inhibitor
Pgp	Dabigatran etexilate, digoxin, fexofenadine	Amiodarone, carvedilol, clarithromycin, dronedarone, itraconazole, lapatinib, lopinavir and ritonavir, propafenone, quinidine, ranolazine, ritonavir, saquinavir and ritonavir, telaprevir, tipranavir and ritonavir, verapamil
BCRP	Rosuvastatin, sulfasalazine	Curcumin, cyclosporine A, eltrombopag
OATP1B1, OATP1B3	Asunaprevir, atorvastatin, bosentan, danoprevir, docetaxel, fexofenadine, glyburide, nateglinide, paclitaxel, pitavastatin, pravastatin, repaglinide, rosuvastatin, simvastatin acid	Atazanavir and ritonavir, clarithromycin, cyclosporine, erythromycin, gemfibrozil, lopinavir and ritonavir, rifampin (single dose), simeprevir
OAT1, OAT3	Adefovir, cefaclor, ceftizoxime, famotidine, furosemide, ganciclovir, methotrexate, oseltamivir carboxylate, penicillin G	*p*-aminohippuric acid (PAH), probenecid, teriflunomide
MATE1, MATE-2 K	Metformin	Cimetidine, dolutegravir, isavuconazole, ranolazine, trimethoprim, vandetanib
OCT2	Metformin	Not available

https://www.fda.gov/drugs/drug-interactions-labeling/drug-development-and-drug-interactions-table-substrates-inhibitors-and-inducers (Accessed on 5-10-2021)

3.6   What Role Does Plasma Protein Binding Play in Drug Discovery?

It is well known that drugs in circulation bind non-covalently to plasma proteins, specifically albumin, α-acid glycoprotein, and less commonly lipoproteins. Acidic and neutral compounds tend to bind to albumin and basic compounds tend to bind to α-acid glycoprotein. The concentration of albumin in blood is very high, about 670 μM, and therefore, it is nearly impossible to saturate binding to albumin. Moreover, albumin has multiple binding pockets. In contrast, the concentration of α-acid glycoprotein is much lower, about 16 μM (but it can be as high as 60 μM in response to inflammation). Therefore, many compounds that bind to α-acid glycoprotein display concentration-dependent plasma protein binding with a larger free fraction at higher concentration. Moreover, α-acid glycoprotein is an active phase protein, which means that it can be up or down regulated as a function of disease state. While plasma protein binding is seemingly a simple concept, it continues to be misinterpreted by many and deserves close attention. While it is an important parameter to know – it is essential to determine the free concentration in either *in vitro* or *in vivo* studies and it is the free concentration that drives the pharmacological effect – it is generally not a parameter that should be 'optimized' (with rare exceptions as described below). In the literature as well as this book, the terms free drug and unbound drug are used interchangeably.

> Plasma protein binding alone cannot be regarded as either a positive or negative aspect of a compound.
>
> Van de Waterbeemd et al. 2001.

The most common method to measure plasma protein binding (PPB) is via equilibrium dialysis. The two compartments of the equilibrium device are separated by a semi-permeable membrane that allows diffusion of small molecules, but not proteins. The plasma resides on one side of the membrane and the buffer is present on the other side. The drug is usually spiked into the plasma side (compartment) and allowed to diffuse across the membrane to the buffer compartment. It usually takes about 6 hours to reach equilibrium, but for compounds with poor physicochemical properties and, hence, low permeability across the semi-permeable membrane, such as zwitter ionic drugs, it may take as long as 24 hours. At the end of the experiment both sides of the equilibrium device are sampled and the concentrations are determined via LC-MS. The unbound or free fraction is determined by the following equation (3.16):

$$f_u = C_u / C_{total} \qquad (3.16)$$

with C_u determined from the buffer side and C_{total} determined from the plasma side of the equilibrium device.

The free fraction allows you to calculate the free drug concentration, which ultimately is usually considered to be responsible for efficacy and toxicity. This is termed the 'free drug hypothesis'. The terms "plasma protein binding" and "free fraction" are used interchangeably, but plasma protein binding refers to the fraction bound to plasma proteins and the free fraction is the inverse, i.e., the fraction not bound to plasma proteins. One of the disadvantages of equilibrium dialysis is non-specific binding to the apparatus. These days, many drug candidates are quite lipophilic and have very small free fractions, < 0.01, and, therefore, the exact free fraction may be hard to determine. New methods have been proposed to address this: (1) dilution of the plasma and pre-saturation to reach equilibrium more quickly (Riccardi et al. 2015) and (2) a bi-directional set up with drug added to either the buffer or plasma side to determine convergence of the free fraction determined either way (Chen et al. 2019).

Ultracentrifugation
Another method to measure plasma protein binding is ultracentrifugation where a centrifuge is used to separate the various components in plasma – such as proteins, lipids and plasma water – in distinct layers, which subsequently can be sampled to determine the free fraction. The top layer contains mainly chylomicrons; the middle layer is the aqueous layer and contains the free drug; the bottom layer is composed of most plasma proteins and, hence, contains the bound drug. Ultracentrifugation is faster than equilibrium dialysis and suffers less from non-specific binding, but has low throughput and the results can be affected by binding to lipoproteins (which reside in the top layer).

Ultrafiltration
Finally, plasma protein binding can be measured via ultrafiltration where two chambers are separated by a semi-permeable membrane with plasma on one side and buffer on the other side. Only the unbound drug crosses the membrane and centrifugation causes separation. Ultrafiltration can also suffer from non-specific binding. Ultracentrifugation and ultrafiltration are less often used because they do not lend themselves to automation very well.

Using the same method, it is also possible to measure tissue binding, such as brain binding, and binding to microsomes. Tissue binding data can be used to determine the local free drug concentration in tissues, which is responsible for driving efficacy and toxicity. Binding to microsomes is an important parameter in the estimation of human clearance from microsomal metabolic stability experiments (see Sect. 6.2.1).

There is a tremendous amount of misconception about the significance of plasma protein binding in the ADME community and, in particular, in the eyes of medicinal chemists. "*Anecdotal collection of publications and presentations would indicate that over one-half of the drug research scientific community has been misled.*"

(Smith and Rowland 2019) Many people think that plasma protein binding needs to be 'optimized' and that a small free fraction is highly undesirable and should be avoided at all cost. The erroneous thinking is that a small free fraction will result in a low free drug concentration, which may not be sufficient to generate an efficacious response. However, there are many successful drugs with very high plasma protein binding, commonly defined as greater than 99%, as shown in Fig. 3.14 – reported plasma protein binding values of drugs approved by the FDA from 2003 to 2016. The proper interpretation of plasma protein binding is covered in a few excellent review articles (Smith et al. 2010; Liu et al. 2011; Liu et al. 2014) and will be summarized here. First, the 'free drug principle' specifies that (1) the pharmacological effect is driven by the unbound drug, i.e. the amount of drug not bound non-specifically to proteins, and (2) the unbound drug is in equilibrium across cell membranes such that $C_{plasma,u} = C_{tissue,u}$ (in the absence of the involvement of drug transporters – see below). Thus, the amount of drug that is unbound in plasma is a good surrogate for the amount unbound in tissues and at the site of action, which may be harder to sample and determine. (The latter can be done in preclinical studies, but may require a large number of animals because each tissue time point is terminal. It is usually impossible to determine in humans although tissue biopsies have become more prevalent in oncology.) If the membrane permeability is low – in the absence of transporters and pH effects as described below – it will obviously take longer to reach steady state, but at steady state the unbound extracellular and intracellular concentration should be roughly equal. The amount of unbound drug in plasma is **solely** determined by the unbound intrinsic hepatic clearance (assuming that clearance is driven by metabolism in the liver and transporters are not involved) and not by the plasma protein binding. Indeed, high plasma protein binding will result in high total drug levels (= unbound drug + bound drug), but will not affect the unbound drug level. Again, the free drug levels are determined by the unbound intrinsic hepatic clearance and not by the plasma protein binding. This is the exact

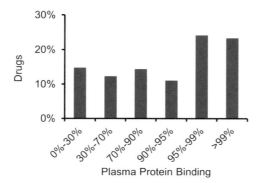

Fig. 3.14 Plasma protein binding of drugs approved by the FDA from 2003 to 2016. (Data from prescription drug labels)

reason why some drugs with high plasma protein binding, such as zelboraf, have high total drug levels in circulation, but still need high doses for efficacy (960 mg twice a day for zelboraf). The total clearance may be low and, hence, the total plasma levels may be high. However, the unbound clearance (CL/f_u) is frequently remarkably high resulting in low free drug levels and, hence, the need for a high dose to reach efficacy.

For highly permeable compounds that are not substrates of transporters, the free concentration in plasma is the same as the free concentration in tissues. The hidden assumption here is that the pH values in plasma and tissue are the same. Exceptions to this rule are tissues rich in lysosomes, which have a much lower pH (pH = 4.5–5); lysosomes are particularly abundant in the lung. In that situation, basic compounds, such as the antimalarial drug chloroquine, will ionize in the lysosomes and the ionized form accumulates in the lysosomes because of its poorly membrane permeability. The unbound concentration of the neutral form of the compound is still the same in plasma and those tissues rich in lysosomes, but the total unbound concentration (unionized + ionized form) is higher in those tissues than plasma because of the accumulation of ionized material at low pH in the lysosomes. This phenomenon is called lysosomal trapping and it is fully reversible. Lysosomal trapping is not applicable to neutral compounds.

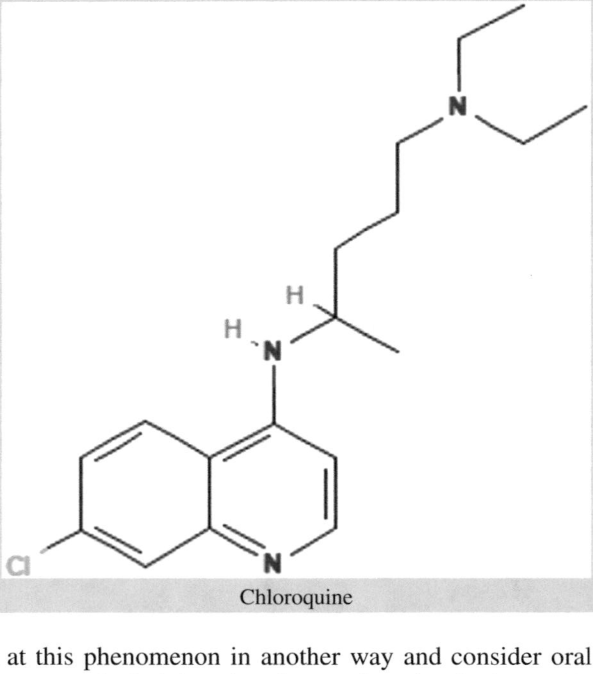

Chloroquine

Let's look at this phenomenon in another way and consider oral dosing – the most common route of administration for small molecule drugs. Usually, it is the total clearance value that is determined and reported in PK reports following intravenous dosing, and frequently it is this parameter that is optimized, i.e., reduced. It may appear that the total clearance can be reduced by increasing the plasma protein binding and reducing f_u (all other things being equal) – see EQ. 3.17a.

$$CL = CL_u \times f_u \tag{3.17a}$$

$$CL_u = CL / f_u \tag{3.17b}$$

However, this is a doomed strategy for a number of reasons. First, CL_u and f_u, while nominally independent parameters, are statistically inversely correlated with lipophilicity; CL_u increases and f_u decreases with increasing lipophilicity and the net effect may be negligible. Second and more importantly, it is the unbound intrinsic clearance that needs to be reduced because it is this parameter that determines the unbound concentration that drives the pharmacology and, therefore, the dose. If we assume for a moment that the efficacious oral dose (as determined by dose fractionation studies) is determined by the average steady state unbound concentration, $C_{avg,ss,u}$, the following equation applies.

$$\text{Dose} = C_{avg,ss,u} \times CL_u \times \tau / F \tag{3.18}$$

$C_{avg,ss,u}$: average steady state unbound concentration and defined here by the *in vitro* potency against the target, e.g. IC_{50} (corrected for any non-specific binding in the incubation); CL_u: human unbound clearance, e.g., derived from human liver microsomes or hepatocytes (corrected for binding in the incubation; directly related to CL_{int}); τ: dosing interval (usually 12 or 24 hours); F: bioavailability.

The above equation assumes that the efficacious oral dose is determined by the average steady state concentration, $C_{avg,ss,u}$, which in turn should be such to provide a certain degree of target coverage (e.g., IC_{50} or, more conservatively, IC_{90}). (Analogous equations can be derived if the dose is determined by the C_{max}, C_{min} or AUC). It is important to note that f_u is **not** present in Eq. 3.18 and, therefore, f_u should not influence the dose and it is the dose that is one of the key parameters that needs to be optimized in drug discovery. This does not mean that f_u is irrelevant. Indeed, the combination of unbound concentration and f_u will determine the total drug concentration and it is the total drug concentration that is usually determined in PK studies. However, the magnitude of f_u will not influence the efficacious dose and, hence, f_u should generally not be 'optimized' (with rare exceptions as described below). Of course, the dose required for efficacy can be reduced by improving the potency of the compound, but the latter may not always be easy as it is governed by the structure-potency relationship.

> The only determinants of unbound steady state exposure are intrinsic clearance and dose
> Harold Boxenbaum.

One final consideration is that lipophilicity is a strong contributor to the extent of plasma protein binding. Generally, higher lipophilicity leads to higher plasma protein binding. In addition, high lipophilicity is correlated with high unbound

As described by Eq. 3.18, plasma protein binding is generally not a parameter that should be 'optimized'. However, there is an interesting and relevant exception to that 'rule': acidic drugs. Literature shows that most acidic drugs have a relatively short half-life and most of the acidic drugs with a longer half-life have very high plasma protein binding (> 99%). The short half-life is usually driven by an extremely low volume of distribution.

$$t_{1/2} = V_d \times 0.693 / CL \tag{3.6}$$

$$V_d = V_p + V_t \left(f_u / f_{ut} \right) \tag{3.7}$$

V_p = volume of plasma
V_t = volume of tissue
f_u = unbound fraction in plasma
f_{ut} = unbound fraction in tissue

For acids, f_u is very small and $f_{ut} > f_u$ and, therefore, the contribution of the V_t term in Eq. 3.5 to the overall volume of distribution is small. The extreme case is $V_d = V_p$ and, therefore, the following equation applies.

$$t_{1/2} = \frac{V_p \times 0.693}{CL} = \frac{V_p \times 0.693}{CL_u \times f_u} \tag{3.19}$$

Thus, if f_u **decreases** and CL_u **stays the same**, the effective half-life will **increase**. It is important not to increase the lipophilicity too much in the process because that will usually increase CL_u and then there may not be a net effect on the half-life. This phenomenon is described in detail in Gardiner et al. 2019.

clearance, which is obviously unfavorable (see Eq. 3.18). Finally, highly lipophilic drugs suffer from poor solubility. Thus, it is wise to avoid highly lipophilic drugs whenever possible.

Let's consider another scenario that is not uncommon in drug discovery. The team has identified two structurally distinct leads, compounds A and B. The free fraction in plasma of compound A is 0.01 and 0.1 for compound B. (The large difference in free fraction suggests that they are not close in chemical analogs.) The potency of compound A based on, for example, a biochemical binding assay is 1 nM, whereas the potency of compound B is 5 nM. Next, the potency is measured in a cellular assay in the presence of serum/plasma. Cellular assays are frequently performed in the presence of some serum/plasma to improve the viability of the cells. It may not be 100% serum or plasma, but let's assume it is in this example. (The same principle applies if it is only 10% serum or plasma.) The potency of compound A in the latter cellular assay is 100 nM, whereas the potency of compound B is 50 nM. Assuming that (a) the permeability of both compounds is good and (b) the cellular read out is similar to that from the biochemical enzymatic or binding assay (i.e. the measured endpoint is not distinct and further downstream) and (c) all other PK properties are equal – including the unbound clearance – except the plasma protein binding, which compound is expected to have a lower dose? Many people will select compound B because it is two-fold more potent in the cellular assay. However, the correct answer in this – albeit somewhat artificial – scenario is compound A. The free fraction of compound A is 0.01 and, therefore, the plasma protein binding caused a 100-fold shift from the biochemical to the cellular assay in the presence of 100% plasma (1 nM → 100 nM). In contrast, the free fraction of compound B is 0.1 and, therefore, the shift going from the biochemical assay to the cellular assay in the presence of 100% plasma is only ten-fold (5 nM → 50 nM). According to the 'free drug hypothesis' – and illustrated in Eq. 3.18 – it is the unbound potency that determines $C_{avg,ss,u}$ (assuming that $C_{avg,ss,u}$ is the driver of efficacy) and ultimately the dose. Thus, assuming that the unbound clearance values for both compounds A and B are the same, the required free drug levels and, hence, the efficacious dose are lower for compound A (see Eq. 3.18) and a lower dose is always advantageous.

In contrast, the total drugs levels at the efficacious dose will be lower for compound B because of the lower plasma protein binding. However, the free drug levels and the corresponding efficacious dose for compound B will be higher. This is graphically depicted in Fig. 3.15.

Cellular potency assays are usually performed in the presence of diluted plasma or serum, usually 5 to 20% to maintain cell viability and function. While this percentage may appear low, a substantial fraction of the compound in the incubation medium may bind to the plasma proteins and any measured potency value, e.g. IC_{50}, may appear artificially high. For example, if the free fraction of a compound in 100% plasma is equal to 0.01, 9% will be free in the presence of 10% plasma. Therefore, it is important to know the plasma protein binding under those conditions to properly interpret the potency data and to distinguish improvements in potency versus a change in plasma protein binding. Plasma protein binding can be either measured in diluted plasma or the following equation can be used to calculate the unbound fraction in diluted plasma.

$$Undiluted\ fu = \frac{1/D}{\left(\left(\frac{1}{fu,d}\right)-1\right)+1/D} \tag{3.20}$$

D = dilution factor
$f_{u,d} = f_u$ in diluted plasma

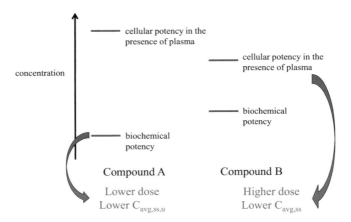

Fig. 3.15 Comparison of biochemical potency and cellular potency (in the presence of plasma) of two compounds (**a** and **b**) and the implications for the unbound and total drug levels as well as the efficacious dose

The publication by Dash et al. 2020 provides additional insight about the interpretation of *in vitro* potency assays.

One final consideration is that lipophilicity is a strong contributor to the extent of plasma protein binding. Generally, a higher lipophilicity leads to higher plasma protein binding. In addition, high lipophilicity is correlated with high unbound clearance.

While the free concentration is the same for drugs that are freely permeable across membranes, the same cannot be said if drug transporters are involved. Uptake transporters, such as OATP1B1 and OATP1B3, are responsible for the uptake of lipophilic acids into the liver (e.g., statins) and, therefore, the free concentration in the liver exceeds that in the plasma. Also, many compounds are substrates of P-glycoprotein and are actively effluxed out of the brain, which results in a much lower free drug concentration in the brain compared to that in the plasma. A complete overview of situations where there is asymmetry between plasma and tissue unbound concentrations is presented in Zhang et al. 2019.

A feature – albeit not new – that has received a lot of attention recently is albumin-mediated uptake. The debate rages on in the ADME community whether the phenomenon is real or an experimental artifact and, if it is real, what the exact mechanism is. However, it appears that the presence of albumin in hepatocytes increases the hepatic uptake of, for example, lipophilic acids, which in turn improves the *in vitro-in vivo* correlation. Some argue that it enhances transporter-mediated hepatic uptake. A detailed overview is beyond the scope of this book and the reader is encouraged to read Bowman and Benet 2018.

3.7   Reactive Metabolites: Bioactivation

Reactive metabolites have been implicated in some cases of toxicity although establishing direct link between reactive metabolites formation and toxicity is complex. The liver is frequently the target organ of reactive metabolites because of the high levels of drug and drug metabolizing enzymes. A well-established example is the severe hepatoxicity associated with bioactivation of acetaminophen to N-acetyl-p-quinoneimine (NAPQI; reactive metabolite) at high doses. After saturating the detoxification conjugative pathways and depleting intracellular glutathione (GSH), NAPQI reacts with critical cellular protein nucleophiles and produces cellular necrosis.

Idiosyncratic Toxicity

An idiosyncratic drug reaction is defined as hypersensitivity to a substance without a direct connection to the pharmacological target of the drug. Although the underlying mechanism is usually unknown, the toxicological response appears to involve direct hepatotoxicity and/or adverse immune reactions. Characteristics of an idiosyncratic drug reaction are:

1. A low incidence (e.g., bromfenac toxicity is seen in 1 out of 20,000 patients).
2. No uniform response from patient to patient.
3. No clear dose/exposure–response relationship. The response is usually more pronounced after repetition of the treatment. An example is Stevens–Johnson syndrome caused by carbamazepine. Note that some patients may be genetically predisposed to such drug reactions, such as those that might carry a specific human leukocyte antigen.

Tools to Assess Bioactivation
- Structural alert
- Trapping reactive metabolites with GSH. There are other trapping agents that capture formation of hard electrophile such as cyanide to trap imines and methoxylamine or semicarbazide for trapping aldehydes.
- Determining the time-dependent inhibition of cytochrome P450 (CYP) enzymes. This is an indirect way to capture potential reactive metabolite formation. The concordance of this versus the first two mentioned above is limited. This in part has to do with different mechanisms that leads to inactivation of CYP enzymes includes reactive oxygen species (ROS) and very short half-life RM that does not escape the active site.

- Assays to determine covalent binding using ^{14}C or ^{3}H labeled compounds from in vitro incubation or in vivo tissues.
- Estimate the contribution of bioactivation pathway(s) to the total elimination pathways
- Monitoring the formation of stable metabolites that points to formation of reactive metabolites such as the detection of carboxylic acids from terminal acetylenes.

Bioactivation in the Context of Drug Discovery

The steps a metabolism scientist should take when bioactivation (defined by formation of GSH or other adducts, covalent binding, or mechanism-based inactivation of CYP enzymes) is observed, continues to be debated in the literature. It is clear that covalent binding can be a liability, but it is not necessarily a showstopper. The following aspects should be taken into consideration:

- Bioactivation should not be a clearance mechanism for a chronically used drug with expected safety margins.
- Understanding the extent of adduct formation, covalent binding or mechanism-based CYP enzyme inactivation in the context of total metabolism.
- Not all *in vitro* observations translate into *in vivo* liabilities because alternative, detoxifying clearance pathways may exist *in vivo*. For example, in the case of raloxifene, *in vitro* incubation with human liver microsomes and nicotinamide adenine dinucleotide phosphate (NADPH) leads to formation of GSH conjugates and covalent binding. However, *in vivo* the main route of elimination for raloxifene is glucuronidation in the intestine and liver (Dalvie et al., 2008).
- A low dose and/or low systemic exposure greatly reduces the risk for serious toxicity.
- Duration of therapy – short term treatment (e.g., antibiotics) versus long term use in relatively healthy patients.
- Therapeutic area – life-threatening diseases versus drug lifestyle drugs (e.g., obesity).
- Target population – some patient populations may be more sensitive to bioactivation than others.
- If a prototype for a new target or compound aims for best-in-class classification.
- Species differences – not all species process drugs the same way, and bioactivation may be unique to one species.

Case 3.19: Moieties that can Result in Reactive Metabolite Formation

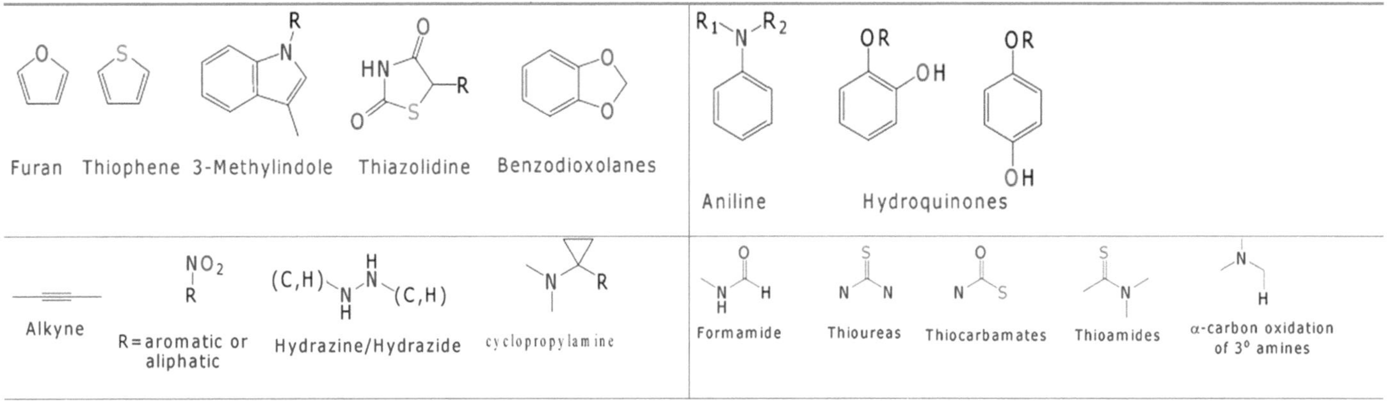

Furan   Thiophene   3-Methylindole   Thiazolidine   Benzodioxolanes

Aniline   Hydroquinones

Alkyne   R=aromatic or   Hydrazine/Hydrazide   cyclopropylamine
         aliphatic

Formamide   Thioureas   Thiocarbamates   Thioamides

α-carbon oxidation
of 3° amines

Case 3.20: Removing Reactive Metabolite

N-Methylcarbamate of CH5447240 was prone to hydrolysis and formation of aniline.

The aniline is further oxidized to form an intermediate that reacts with GSH at the benzylic position.

Replacement with 5,5-dimethylhydantoin removes the hydrolytic liability for formatting the aniline (Nishimura et al. 2020).

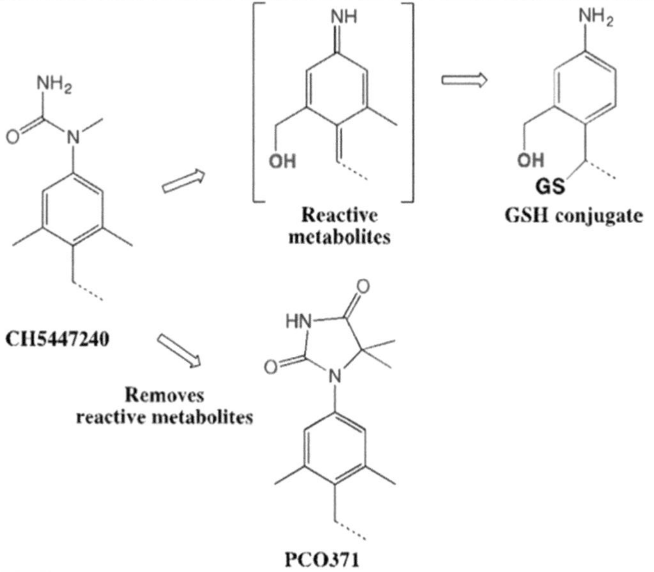

Reactive metabolites

GSH conjugate

CH5447240

Removes reactive metabolites

PCO371

Case 3.21: Isosteres of Aminothiazole to Fix Reactive Metabolites Formation

Optimization for removing aminothiazole (a structural alerts) by replacing with changing positon of thiol plus intorducing another nitrogen atom (thiodiazole) for the discovery of PF-05089771.

Target: selective NaV1.7 inhibitors

Swain et al. 2017

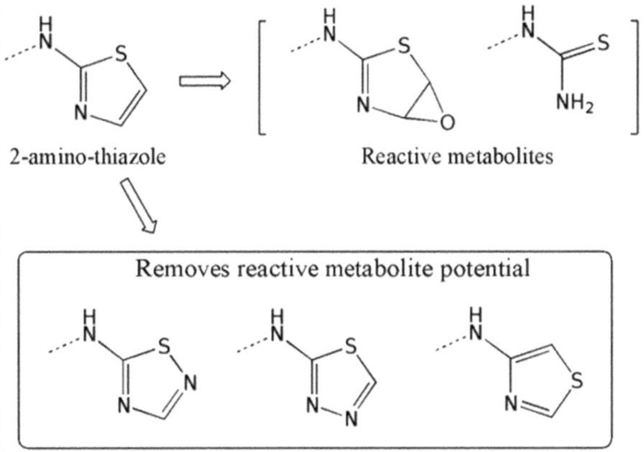

Case 3.22: Using of Metabolic Switching to Remove Reactive Metabolites

Bioactivation was observed due to reactive metabolite formation
likely at urea moiety which is critical for potency.

Other parts of the molecule was changed to result in metabolic
switching (new soft spot) that took the metabolism away from the
urea moiety. As a result, a negligible formation of reactive
metabolite was formed (Grillot et al. 2014).

Target: Gram-positive anti-bacterial activity.

Case 3.23: Mechanisms of Bioactivation

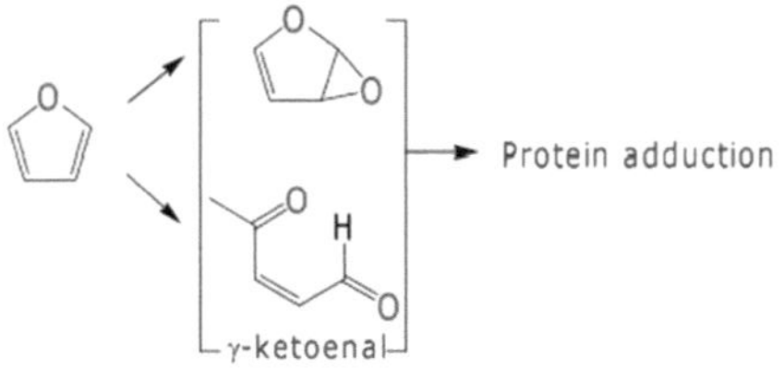

ipomeanol, furosemide, menthofuran, aflatoxin B1

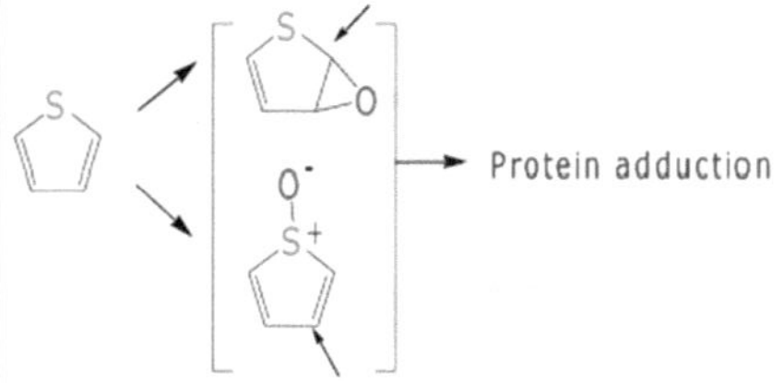

Tienilic acid, Suprofen, Ticlopidine, Tenoxicam

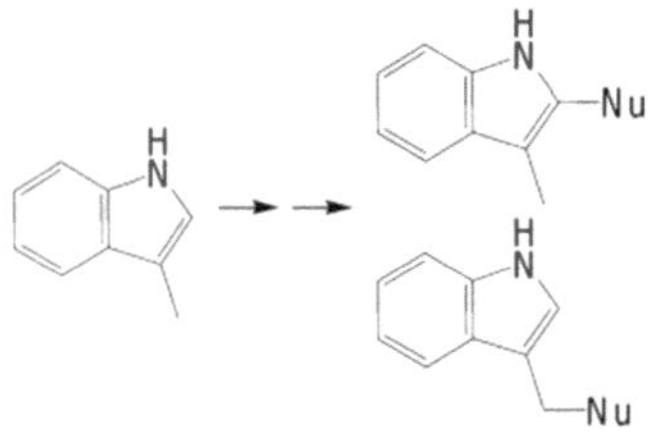

Acetaminophen, amodiaquine, dichlophenac

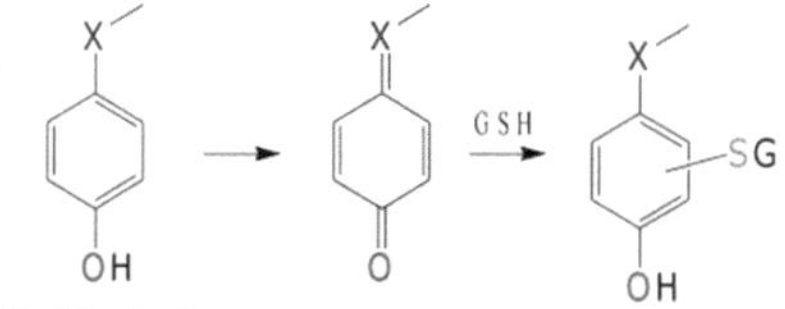

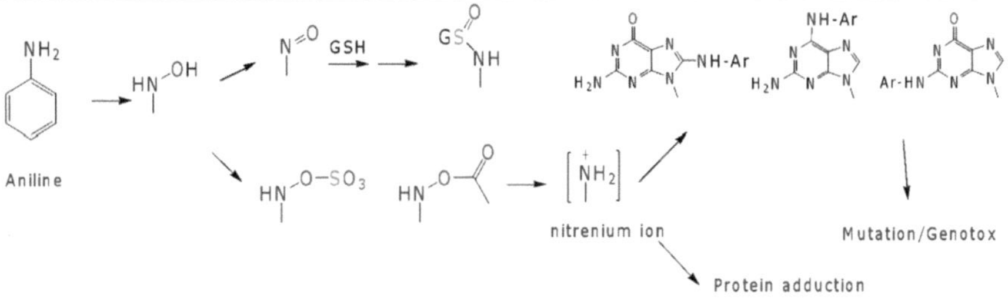

L-745,870

Procainamide, sulfamethoxazole, dapsone

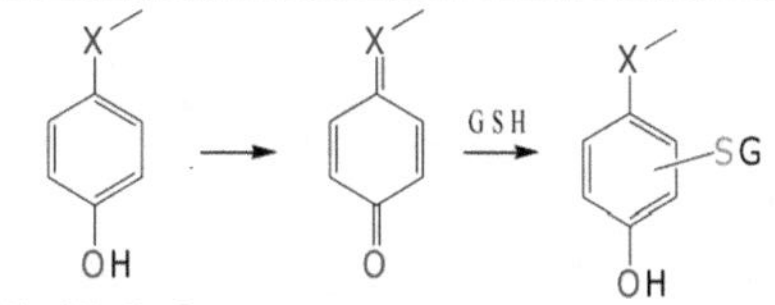

X = CH, N, O

GSH

Acetaminophen, amodiaquine, dichlophenac

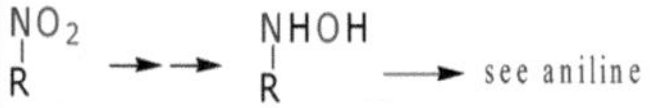

Thiazolidine

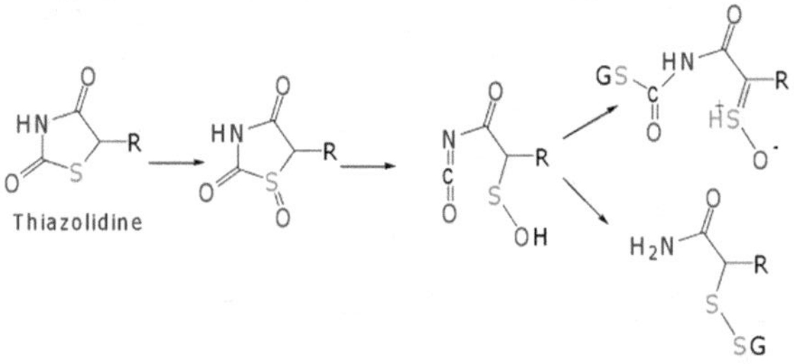

Troglitazone, rosiglitazone, pioglitazone

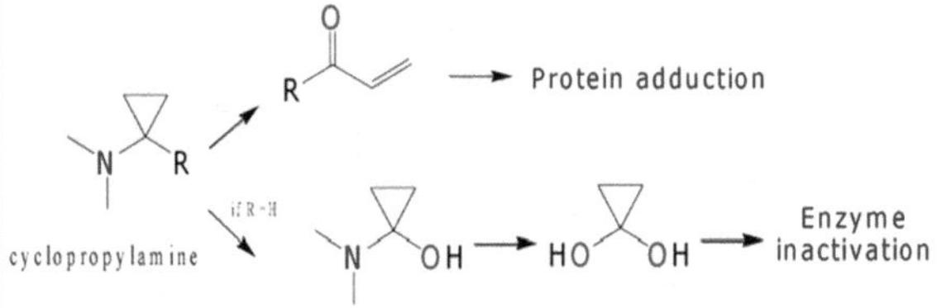

α-carbon oxidation of 3° amines

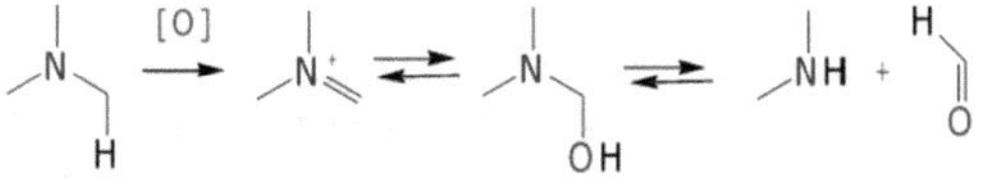

[O]

Pyrrolidine, piperidine, N-mehtylpyrrole, morpholine ring

NO_2 NHOH   see aniline

4-nitroquinoline-1-oxide, Nitrofurazone, nitrofurantoin

Protein adduction

Enzyme inactivation

cyclopropylamine

3.8   Supplemental Materials

Table 3.S.1   Phase I drug metabolizing enzymes and their subcellular location or blood

Pathway	Enzyme (abbreviation) EC number	Subcellular location or blood
Oxidation	Alcohol dehydrogenase (ADH) 1.1.1	Cytosol, blood vessels
	Aldehyde dehydrogenase (ALDH) 1.2.1	Mitochondria, cytosol
	Aldehyde oxidase (AO) 1.2.3.1	Cytosol
	Aldo-keto reductase (AKR)	Cytosol
	Cytochrome P450 (P450 or CYP) 1.14.13 & 1.14.14.1	ER
	Diamine oxidase (DAO) 1.4.3.6	Cytosol
	Flavin-containing monooxygenase (FMO) 1.14.13.8	ER
	Monoamine oxidase (MAO) 1.4.3.4	Mitochondria
	Prostaglandin H synthase (PGHS) 1.14.99.1	ER
	Xanthine oxidase/xanthine dehydrogenase (XO/XDH) 1.2.3.2/1.17.1.4	Cytosol
Hydrolysis	Carboxylesterase (CE) 3.1.1.1	ER, cytosol, lysosome
	Epoxide hydrolase (EH) 3.3.2	ER, cytosol
	β-Glucuronidase 3.2.1.31	Lysosomes, ER, blood, gut bacteria
	Arylesterases/Paraoxonases (PON) 3.1.1.2	
	Pseudocholinesterase/Butyrylcholinesterase (BuChE) 3.1.1.8	Cytosol
	Peptidase	Blood, lysosomes
Reduction	Azo- and nitro-reductase	Microflora, ER, cytosol
	Carbonyl reductase	Cytosol, blood, ER
	Disulfide reductase	Cytosol
	Quinone reductase (NQO) 1.6.5.5	Cytosol, ER
	Sulfoxide reductase	Cytosol
	Reductive dehydrogenase	ER

EC enzyme classification, *ER* endoplasmic reticulum

Table 3.S.2   Phase II drug metabolizing enzymes and subcellular location or blood

Enzyme (abbreviation) EC number	Subcellular location or blood
Uridine diphosphate glucuronosyltransferase (UGT) 2.4.1.17	ER
Sulfotransferase (SULT) 2.8.2	Cytosol
Glutathione transferase (GST) 2.5.1.18	Cytosol, ER
Amino acid conjugate systems	Mitochondria, ER
N-acetyl transferase (NAT) 2.3.1.87	Cytosol
Methyltransferases	Cytosol, ER, blood

EC enzyme number, *ER* endoplasmic reticulum

Table 3.S.3 Major CYP isoforms in different species

Isoform	Mouse	Rat	Dog	Monkey	Human
CYP1	1a1, 1a2, 1b1	1A1, 1A2, 1B1	1A1, 1A2, 1B1	1A1, 1A2, 1B1	1A1, 1A2, 1B1
CYP2A	2a4, 2a5, 2a12, 2A22	2A1, 2A2, 2A3	2A13, 2A25	2A23, 2A23	2A6, 2A7, 2A13
CYP2B	2b9, 2b10	2B1, 2B2, 2B3	2B11	2B17	2B6, 2B7
CYP2C	2c29, 2c37, 2c38, 2c39, 2c40, 2c44, 2c50, 2c54, 2c55	2C6, 2C7, 2C11[a], 2C12[a], 2C13[a], 2C22, 2C23	2C21, 2C41[b]	2C20, 2C43	2C8, 2C9, 2C18, 2C19
CYP2D	2d9, 2d10, 2d11, 2d12, 2d13, 2d22, 2d26, 2d34, 2d40	2D1, 2D2, 2D3, 2D4, 2D5, 2D18	2D15	2D17, 2D19, 2D29, 2D30	2D6, 2D7, 2D8
CYP2E	2e1	2E1	2E1	2E1	2E1
CYP3A	3a11[c], 3a13, 3a16, 3a25, 3a41, 3a44	3A1/3A23, 3A2[d], 3A9[d], 3A9, 3A18[d], 3A62	3A12, 3A26	3A8[e]	3A4, 3A5, 3A7[f], 3A43

Martignoni et al. (2006)

Note that mouse isoforms are written in lower case

[a]CYP2C11 is male specific and is 50% of the total CYP concentration in male rats. CYP2C12 is female adult specific. CYP2C13 is male specific

[b]CYP2C41 is homologous with human CYP2Cs

[c]The highest activity of 3a11 is seen at 4–8 weeks of age

[d]CYP3A2 and 3A18 are male specific and CYP3A9 is female specific

[e]CYP3A8 is 20% of the total concentration of monkey hepatic CYP isoforms

[f]CYP3A7 is only highly expressed in infants

References

Ahlström MM, Ridderström M, Zamora I (2007) CYP2C9 structure−metabolism relationships: substrates, inhibitors, and metabolites. J Med Chem 50(22):5382–5391. https://doi.org/10.1021/jm070745g

Akabane T, Tanaka K, Irie M, Terashita S, Teramura T (2011) Case report of extensive metabolism by aldehyde oxidase in humans: pharmacokinetics and metabolite profile of FK3453 in rats, dogs, and humans. Xenobiotica 41(5):372–384. https://doi.org/10.3109/0049825 4.2010.549970

Aliagas I, Gobbi A, Heffron T, Lee ML, Ortwine DF, Zak M, Khojasteh SC (2015) A probabilistic method to report predictions from a human liver microsomes stability QSAR model: a practical tool for drug discovery. J Comput Aided Mol Des 29(4):327–338. https://doi.org/10.1007/s10822-015-9838-3. Epub 2015 Feb 24

Balani SK, Zhu T, Yang TJ, Liu Z, He B, Lee FW (2002) Effective dosing regimen of 1-aminobenzotriazole for inhibition of antipyrine clearance in rats, dogs, and monkeys. Drug Metab Dispos 30(10):1059–1062. https://doi.org/10.1124/dmd.30.10.1059

Berry LM, Liu J, Colletti A, Krolikowski P, Zhao Z, Teffera Y (2014) Species difference in glucuronidation formation kinetics with a selective mTOR inhibitor. Drug Metab Dispos 42(4):707–717. https://doi.org/10.1124/dmd.113.054809

Bhhatarai B, Walters WP, Hop CECA et al (2019) Opportunities and challenges using artificial intelligence in ADME/Tox. Nature Mater 18(5):418–422

Bolleddula J, DeMent K, Driscoll JP, Worboys P, Brassil PJ, Bourdet DL (2014) Biotransformation and bioactivation reactions of alicyclic amines in drug molecules. Drug Metab Rev 46(3):379–419. https://doi.org/10.3109/03602532.2014.924962

Bowman CM, Benet LZ (2018) An examination of protein binding and protein-facilitated uptake relating to *in vitro-in vivo* extrapolation. Eur J Pharm Sci 123:502–514

Boxenbaum H, Battle M (1995) Effective half-life in clinical pharmacology. J Clin Pharmacol 35:763–766

Broccatelli F, Hop M, Wright M (2019) Strategies to optimize drug half-life in lead candidate identification. Expert Opin Drug Dis 14(3):221–230. https://doi.org/10.1080/1746044 1.2019.1569625

Brouwer KLR, Keppler D, Hoffmaster KA et al (2013) In vitro methods to support transporter evaluation in drug discovery and development. Clin Pharmacol Ther 94(1):95–112. https://doi.org/10.1038/clpt.2013.81

Brown et al (1997) Physiological parameter values for physiologically based pharmacokinetics models. Toxicol Ind Health 13(4):407–484

Chen Y-C, Kenny JR, Wright M, Hop CECA, Yan Z (2019) Improving confidence in the determination of free fraction for highly bound drugs using bidirectional equilibrium dialysis. J Pharm Sci 108(3):1296–1302

Cheng Y, Wang L, Iacono L et al (2018) Clinical significance of CYP2C19 polymorphisms on the metabolism and pharmacokinetics of 11β-hydroxysteroid dehydrogenase Type-1 inhibitor BMS-823778. Brit J Clin Pharmaco 84(1):130–141. https://doi.org/10.1111/bcp.13421

Cruciani G, Valeri A, Goracci L, Pellegrino RM, Buonerba F, Baroni M (2014) Flavin monooxygenase metabolism: why medicinal chemists should matter. J Med Chem 57(14):6183–6196. https://doi.org/10.1021/jm5007098

Dahal UP, Joswig-Jones C, Jones J (2011) Comparative study of the affinity and metabolism of type I and type II binding quinoline carboxamide analogues by cytochrome P450 3A4. J Med Chem 55(1):280–290. https://doi.org/10.1021/jm201207h

Dalvie D, Kang P, Zientek M, Xiang C, Zhou S, Obach RS (2008) Effect of intestinal glucuronidation in limiting hepatic exposure and bioactivation of raloxifene in humans and rats. Chem Res Toxicol 21(12):2260–2271. https://doi.org/10.1021/tx800323w

Dash RP, Thomas JA, Rosenfeld C, Srinivas NR (2020) Protein binding and stability of drug candidates: the Achilles' heel of *in vitro* potency assays. Eur J Drug Metab Pharmacokinet 45(4):427–432

Davies B, Morris T (1993) Physiological parameters in laboratory animals and humans. Pharm Res 10:1093–1095

de Montellano PRO (2018) 1-Aminobenzotriazole: a mechanism-based cytochrome P450 inhibitor and probe of cytochrome P450 biology. Med Chem 8(3):38–65. https://doi.org/10.4172/2161-0444.1000495

Diamond S, Boer J, Maduskuie TP, Falahatpisheh N, Li Y, Yeleswaram S (2010) Species-specific metabolism of SGX523 by aldehyde oxidase and the toxicological implications. Drug Metab Dispos 38(8):1277–1285. https://doi.org/10.1124/dmd.110.032375

El-Kattan AF, Varma MVS (2018) Navigating transporter sciences in pharmacokinetics characterization using extended clearance classification system (ECCS). Drug Metab Dispos 46(5):dmd.117.080044. https://doi.org/10.1124/dmd.117.080044

Fan PW, Zhang D, Halladay JS, Driscoll JP, Khojasteh SC (2016) Going beyond common drug metabolizing enzymes: case studies of biotransformation involving aldehyde oxidase, γ-glutamyl transpeptidase, cathepsin b, flavin-containing monooxygenase, and ADP-ribosyltransferase. Drug Metab Dispos 44(8):1253–1261. https://doi.org/10.1124/dmd.116.070169

Farooq M, Kelly EJ, Unadkat JD (2016) CYP2D6 is inducible by endogenous and exogenous corticosteroids. Drug Metab Dispos 44(5):750–757. https://doi.org/10.1124/dmd.115.069229. (Retraction published Drug Metab Dispos 2018 Sep;46(9):1360)

Gardiner P, Cox RJ, Grime K (2019) Plasma protein binding as an optimizable parameter for acidic drugs. Drug Metab Dispos 47(8):865–873

Ghosh AK, Brindisi M (2019) Urea derivatives in modern drug discovery and medicinal chemistry. J Med Chem 63(6):2751–2788. https://doi.org/10.1021/acs.jmedchem.9b01541

Grillot AL, Le Tiran A, Shannon D, Krueger E, Liao Y, O'Dowd H, Tang Q, Ronkin S, Wang T, Waal N, Li P, Lauffer D, Sizensky E, Tanoury J, Perola E, Grossman TH, Doyle T, Hanzelka B, Jones S, Dixit V, Ewing N, Liao S, Boucher B, Jacobs M, Bennani Y, Charifson PS (2014) Second-generation antibacterial benzimidazole ureas: discovery of a preclinical candidate with reduced metabolic liability. J Med Chem 57(21):8792–8816. https://doi.org/10.1021/jm500563g. Epub 2014 Oct 28

He K, Qian M, Wong H et al (2008) N-in-1 dosing pharmacokinetics in drug discovery- Experience, theoretical and practical considerations. J Pharm Sci, 97:2568–2580

Jones JP, Korzekwa KR (2013) Predicting intrinsic clearance for drugs and drug candidates metabolized by aldehyde oxidase. Mol Pharm 10(4):1262–1268. https://doi.org/10.1021/mp300568r

Kempf DJ, Sham HL, Marsh KC et al (1998) Discovery of ritonavir, a potent inhibitor of HIV protease with high oral bioavailability and clinical efficacy. J Med Chem 41(4):602–617. https://doi.org/10.1021/jm970636+

Kumari A, Singh RK (2020) Morpholine as ubiquitous pharmacophore in medicinal chemistry: deep insight into the structure-activity relationship (SAR). Bioorg Chem 96:103578. https://doi.org/10.1016/j.bioorg.2020.103578

Lassalas P, Gay B, Lasfargeas C et al (2016) Structure property relationships of carboxylic acid isosteres. J Med Chem 59(7):3183–3203. https://doi.org/10.1021/acs.jmedchem.5b01963

Lentz KA, Quitko M, Morgan DG et al (2007) Development and validation of a preclinical food effect model. J Pharm Sci 96:459–472

Liu B, Chang J, Gordon WP, Isbell J, Zhou Y, Tuntland T (2008) Snapshot PK: a rapid rodent in vivo preclinical screening approach. Drug Discov Today 13:360–367

Liu X, Chen C, Hop CECA (2011) Do we need to optimize plasma protein and tissue binding in drug discovery? Curr Top Med Chem 11(4):450–466

Liu X, Ding X, Deshmukh G, Liederer BM, Hop CECA (2012) Use of the cassette-dosing approach to assess brain penetration in drug discovery. Drug Metab Dispos 40:963–969

Liu X, Wright M, Hop CECA (2014) Rational use of plasma protein and tissue binding data in drug design. J Med Chem 57(20):8238–8248

Lolkema MP, Bohets HH, Arkenau H-T et al (2015) The c-met tyrosine kinase inhibitor JNJ-38877605 causes renal toxicity through species-specific insoluble metabolite formation. Clin Cancer Res 21(10):2297–2304. https://doi.org/10.1158/1078-0432.ccr-14-3258

Lombardo F, Desai PV, Arimoto R et al (2017) In silico absorption, distribution, metabolism, excretion, and pharmacokinetics (ADME-PK): utility and best practices. An industry perspective from the international consortium for innovation through quality in pharmaceutical development. J Med Chem 60(22):9097–9113

Manevski N, King L, Pitt WR, Lecomte F, Toselli F (2019) Metabolism by aldehyde oxidase: drug design and complementary approaches to challenges in drug discovery. J Med Chem 62(24):10955–10994. https://doi.org/10.1021/acs.jmedchem.9b00875

Martignoni M, Groothuis GM, de Kanter R (2006) Species differences between mouse, rat, dog, monkey and human CYP-mediated drug metabolism, inhibition and induction. Expert Opin Drug Metab Toxicol 2(6):875–894. https://doi.org/10.1517/17425255.2.6.875

Mei H, Korfmacher W, Morrison R (2006) Rapid in vivo oral screening in rats: reliability, acceptance criteria, and filtering efficiency. AAPS J 8:E493–E500

Meschter CL, Mico BA, Mortillo M et al (1994) A 13-week toxicologic and pathologic evaluation of prolonged cytochromes p450 inhibition by 1-aminobenzotriazole in male rats. Fund Appl Toxicol 22(3):369–381. https://doi.org/10.1006/faat.1994.1042

Morgan P, Brown DG, Lennard S et al (2018) Impact of a five-dimensional framework on R & D productivity at AstraZeneca. Nature Rev Drug Discov 17(3):167–181

Morisseau C, Hammock BD (2005) Epoxide hydrolases: mechanisms, inhibitor designs, and biological roles. Annu Rev Pharmacol Toxicol 45:311–333. https://doi.org/10.1146/annurev. pharmtox.45.120403.095920

Nishimura Y, Esaki T, Isshiki Y et al (2020) Lead optimization and avoidance of reactive metabolite leading to PCO371, a potent, selective, and orally available human parathyroid hormone receptor 1 (HPTHR1) agonist. J Med Chem 63(10):5089–5099. https://doi.org/10.1021/acs. jmedchem.9b01743

Ogilvie BW, Zhang D, Li W et al (2006) Glucuronidation converts gemfibrozil to a potent, metabolism-dependent inhibitor of CYP2C8: implications for drug-drug interactions. Drug Metab Dispos 34(1):191–197. https://doi.org/10.1124/dmd.105.007633

Paine MF, Hart HL, Ludington SS et al (2006) The human intestinal cytochrome P450 "PIE". Drug Metab Dispos 34(5):880–886. https://doi.org/10.1124/dmd.105.008672

Pei Z, Mendonca R, Gazzard L et al (2018) Aminoisoxazoles as potent inhibitors of tryptophan 2,3-dioxygenase 2 (TDO2). ACS Med Chem Lett 9(5):417–421. https://doi.org/10.1021/ acsmedchemlett.7b00427

Rendic S, Carlo FJD (2010) Human cytochrome P450 enzymes: a status report summarizing their reactions, substrates, inducers, and inhibitors. Drug Metab Rev 29(1–2):413–580. https://doi. org/10.3109/03602539709037591

Riccardi K, Cawley S, Yates PD et al (2015) Plasma protein binding of challenging compounds. J Pharm Sci 104(8):2627–2636

Rohde JJ, Pliushchev MA, Sorensen BK (2007) Discovery and metabolic stabilization of potent and selective 2-amino- N -(adamant-2-Yl) acetamide 11β-hydroxysteroid dehydrogenase type 1 inhibitors. J Med Chem 50(1):149–164. https://doi.org/10.1021/jm0609364

Rostami-Hodjegan A, Tucker GT (2007) Simulation and prediction of in vivo drug metabolism in human populations from in vitro data. Nat Rev Drug Discov 6(2):140–148. https://doi. org/10.1038/nrd2173

Siegrist R, Pozzi D, Jacob G et al (2016) Structure–Activity Relationship, drug metabolism and pharmacokinetics properties optimization, and in vivo studies of new brain penetrant triple T-Type calcium channel blockers. J Med Chem 59(23):10661–10675. https://doi.org/10.1021/ acs.jmedchem.6b01356

Smith DA, Rowland M (2019) Intracellular and intraorgan concentrations of small molecule drugs: theory, uncertainties in infectious disease and oncology, and promise. Drug Metab Dispos 47(6):665–672

Smith DA, Di L, Kerns EH (2010) The effect of plasma protein binding on in vivo drug discovery: misconceptions in drug discovery. Nature Rev Drug Discov 9(12):929–939

Smith DA, Beaumont K, Maurer TS, Di L (2018) Clearance in drug design: miniperspective. J Med Chem 62(5):2245–2255. https://doi.org/10.1021/acs.jmedchem.8b01263

Sodhi JK, Ford KA, Mukadam S et al (2014) 1-Aminobenzotriazole coincubated with (S)-warfarin results in potent inactivation of CYP2C9. Drug Metab Dispos 42(5):813–817. https://doi. org/10.1124/dmd.113.055913

Sodhi JK, Wong S, Kirkpatrick DS et al (2015) A novel reaction mediated by human aldehyde oxidase: amide hydrolysis of GDC-0834. Drug Metab Dispos 43(6):908–915. https://doi. org/10.1124/dmd.114.061804

Stearns RA, Miller RR, Tang W et al (2002) The pharmacokinetics of a thiazole benzenesulfonamide beta 3-adrenergic receptor agonist and its analogs in rats, dogs, and monkeys: improving oral bioavailability. Drug Metab Dispos 30(7):771–777. https://doi.org/10.1124/dmd.30.7.771

Stepan AF, Mascitti V, Beaumont K, Kalgutkar AS (2012) Metabolism-guided drug design Medchemcomm 4(4):631–652. https://doi.org/10.1039/c2md20317k

Strelevitz TJ, Foti RS, Fisher MB (2006) In vivo use of the P450 inactivator 1-aminobenzotriazole in the rat: varied dosing route to elucidate gut and liver contributions to first-pass and systemic clearance. J Pharm Sci 95(6):1334–1341. https://doi.org/10.1002/jps.20538

Stringer RA, Weber E, Tigani B, Lavan P, Medhurst S, Sohal B (2014) 1-aminobenzotriazole modulates oral drug pharmacokinetics through cytochrome p450 inhibition and delay of gastric emptying in rats. Drug Metab Dispos 42(7):1117–1124. https://doi.org/10.1124/dmd.113.056408

Sturino CF, O'Neill G, Lachance N et al (2007) Discovery of a potent and selective prostaglandin d 2 receptor antagonist, [(3 r)-4-(4-chloro- benzyl)-7-fluoro-5-(methylsulfonyl)-1,2,3,4-tetrahydrocyclopenta[b]indol-3-yl]-acetic acid (MK-0524). J Med Chem 50(4):794–806. https://doi.org/10.1021/jm0603668

Swain NA, Batchelor D, Beaudoin S, Bechle BM, Bradley PA, Brown AD, Brown B, Butcher KJ, Butt RP, Chapman ML, Denton S, Ellis D, Galan SRG, Gaulier SM, Greener BS, de Groot MJ, Glossop MS, Gurrell IK, Hannam J, Johnson MS, Lin Z, Markworth CJ, Marron BE, Millan DS, Nakagawa S, Pike A, Printzenhoff D, Rawson DJ, Ransley SJ, Reister SM, Sasaki K, Storer RI, Stupple PA, West CW (2017) Discovery of clinical candidate 4-[2-(5-amino-1H-pyrazol-4-yl)-4-chlorophenoxy]-5-chloro-2-fluoro-N-1,3-thiazol-4-ylbenzenesulfonamide (PF-05089771): design and optimization of Diaryl ether aryl Sulfonamides as selective inhibitors of NaV1.7. J Med Chem 60(16):7029–7042. https://doi.org/10.1021/acs.jmedchem.7b00598

The International Transporter Consortium (2010) Membrane Transporters in Drug Development. Nat Rev Drug Discov 9:215–236

Toselli F, Fredenwall M, Svensson P et al (2017) Oxetane substrates of human microsomal epoxide hydrolase. Drug Metab Dispos 45(8):966-973. dmd.117.076489. https://doi.org/10.1124/dmd.117.076489

Uchaipichat V, Mackenzie PI, Elliot DJ, Miners JO (2006) Selectivity of substrate (trifluoperazine) and inhibitor (amitriptyline, androsterone, canrenoic acid, hecogenin, phenylbutazone, quinidine, quinine, and sulfinpyrazone) "probes" for human UDP-glucuronosyltransferases. Drug Metab Dispos 34(3):449–456. https://doi.org/10.1124/dmd.105.007369

Van de Waterbeemd H, Smith DA, Beaumont K, Walker DK (2001) Property-based design: optimization of drug absorption and pharmacokinetics. J Med Chem 44(9):1313–1333

Victor F, Brown TJ, Campanale K et al (1997) Synthesis, antiviral activity, and biological properties of vinylacetylene analogs of enviroxime. J Med Chem 40(10):1511–1518. https://doi.org/10.1021/jm960718i

Watanabe A, Mayumi K, Nishimura K, Osaki H (2016) In vivo use of the CYP inhibitor 1-aminobenzotriazole to increase long-term exposure in mice. Biopharm Drug Dispos 37(6):373–378. https://doi.org/10.1002/bdd.2020

Williams JA, Hyland R, Jones BC et al (2004) Drug-drug interactions for udp-glucuronosyltransferase substrates: a pharmacokinetic explanation for typically observed low exposure (AUCI/AUC) RATIOS. Drug Metab Dispos 32(11):1201–1208. https://doi.org/10.1124/dmd.104.000794

Wong PC, Pinto DJP, Zhang D (2011) Preclinical discovery of apixaban, a direct and orally bioavailable factor Xa inhibitor. J Thromb Thrombolys 31(4):478–492. https://doi.org/10.1007/s11239-011-0551-3

Wu Y-J, Davis CD, Dworetzky S et al (2003) Fluorine substitution can block cyp3a4 metabolism-dependent inhibition: identification of (s) -n -[1-(4-fluoro-3- morpholin-4-ylphenyl)ethyl]-3-(4-fluorophenyl)acrylamide as an orally bioavailable kcnq2 opener devoid of CYP3A4 metabolism-dependent inhibition. J Med Chem 46(18):3778–3781. https://doi.org/10.1021/jm034111v

Xu H, Murray M, McLachlan A (2009) Influence of genetic polymorphisms on the pharmacokinetics and pharmacodynamics of sulfonylurea drugs. Curr Drug Metab 10(6):643–658. https://doi.org/10.2174/138920009789375388

Xu Y, Li L, Wang Y et al (2017) Aldehyde oxidase mediated metabolism in drug-like molecules: a combined computational and experimental study. J Med Chem 60(7):2973–2982. https://doi.org/10.1021/acs.jmedchem.7b00019

Zhang X, Liu H-H, Weller P et al (2011) In Silico and in vitro Pharmacogenetics: aldehyde oxidase rapidly metabolizes a P38 kinase inhibitor. Pharmacogenomics J 11(1):15–24. https://doi.org/10.1038/tpj.2010.8

Zhang D, Hop CECA, Patilea-Vrana G et al (2019) Drug concentration asymmetry in tissues and plasma for small molecule–related therapeutic modalities. Drug Metab Dispos 47(10):1122–1135

Chapter 4
Candidate Translational Characterization

Contents

© Springer Nature Switzerland AG 2022
S. C. Khojasteh et al., *Discovery DMPK Quick Guide*,
https://doi.org/10.1007/978-3-031-10691-0_4

Abstract Promising clinical candidates undergo extensive translational character-ization prior to advancement into activities required for first-in-human clinical tri-als. Translational characterization involves activities such as the prediction of human pharmacokinetics, human dose prediction using PK/PD modeling; predic-tion of human safety margins; and physiologically-based pharmacokinetic model-ing to assess DDI risk. These activities leverage available preclinical data and mathematical modeling in order to provide an early assessment of clinical risk. This chapter introduces activities involved in candidate translational characterization.

Keywords Prediction · Human pharmacokinetics · Dose · Pharmacokinetic · Physiologically-based pharmacokinetic models · Toxicokinetics · Safety margins

Abbreviations

ADME	Absorption, distribution, metabolism and excretion
AUC	Area under the concentration time curve
BrW	Brain weight
$CL_{hepatic}$	Hepatic clearance
CL_{int}	Intrinsic clearance
CL_u	Unbound clearance
C_{max}	The highest concentration that is observed
CYP	cytochrome P450
F	Bioavailability
F_a	Fraction absorbed from the intestine
F_g	Fraction that escapes intestinal metabolism
F_h	Fraction that escapes hepatic metabolism
f_u	Unbound fraction in blood/plasma
f_{umic}	Unbound fraction in microsomes
f_{ut}	Unbound fraction in tissues
HPGL	Hepatocytes per gram of liver
IC_{50}	Concentration at which there is 50% inhibition
IC_{90}	Concentration at which there is 90% inhibition
IVIVE	*In vitro–In vivo* extrapolation
K_m	Michaelis–Menten constant (i.e. substrate concentration when v is ½ of V_{max})
MLP	Maximum life span
MPPGL	Microsomal protein per gram of liver
MRT	Mean residence time
PBPK	Physiologically-based pharmacokinetic model
PK	Pharmacokinetic
PK/PD	Pharmacokinetic/pharmacodynamic
$P_{microsome}$	Amount of microsomal protein in the incubation
Q	Hepatic blood flow
R_e/I	Ratio of binding proteins in extracellular fluid (except plasma) to binding proteins in plasma

$t_{1/2}$	Half-life
$t_{1/2(in\ vitro)}$	*In vitro* half-life
t_{max}	The time that C_{max} is observed
V_d	Volume of distribution
$V_{d,u}$	Unbound volume of distribution
V_e	Extracellular fluid volume
$V_{incubation}$	Incubation volume
V_{max}	Maximum rate of the metabolic reaction
V_p	Plasma volume
V_r	'Remainder' of the fluid volume

4.1   Basic Concepts

The process of translational characterization of a clinical candidate involves attempting to understand how the candidate compound will behave in humans based on the available preclinical data. Figure 4.1 illustrates the process of preclinical translational characterization. Two common objectives for this exercise include assessment of a pharmacological active dose and assessment of safety in humans. Central to these two objectives involves an early assessment of anticipated drug exposures in humans following candidate administration.

The assessment of anticipated drug exposure involves first the prediction of human pharmacokinetics and pharmacokinetic/pharmacodynamic (PK/PD) modeling. The human pharmacokinetic prediction enables the assessment of human drug exposure at various doses. Methodologies that are used in pharmacokinetic

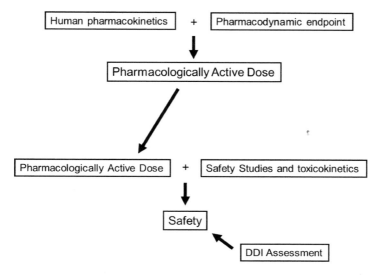

Fig. 4.1 Process of preclinical translational characterization of a drug candidate

prediction are described in later sections of this chapter. PK/PD modeling serves to link anticipated human pharmacokinetics to active drug concentrations and an associated pharmacodynamic endpoint in order to provide both an anticipated pharmacologically active dose in humans as well as efficacious exposures in humans. The identified efficacious exposures serve to provide a reference point from which safety margins and liabilities such as drug-drug interactions (DDI) are assessed.

4.2   Prediction of Human Pharmacokinetics

The prediction of human pharmacokinetics of a clinical candidate is a core activity during the translational characterization of a clinical candidate. Despite the uncertainty of human PK predictions, this activity has led to the reduction of clinical candidate failure due to poor human PK (Kola and Landis 2004). Assessments of human pharmacokinetics can be broadly divided into two categories. Those methods that that rely on in vivo animal PK studies those that rely on in vitro studies.

4.2.1   Human PK Prediction Based on In Vivo Preclinical PK Studies

Methods of predicting human pharmacokinetics relying on *in vivo* PK studies make the assumption that there is some similarity between animals and humans in their ability to clear compounds for predictions of clearance or distribute compounds for predictions of volume of distribution. Many of the *in vivo* methods of prediction of human pharmacokinetics are based on allometry or allometric principles. Allometry in its most basic form assumes a relationship between the human PK parameter of interest and body weight. The equation for simple allometry is as follows:

$$Y = a \times W^b \qquad (4.1)$$

Y = pharmacokinetic parameter; a = coefficient of allometric eq; W = body weight; b = exponent of allometric equation

4.2.2   Simple Allometry for Prediction of Human CL

For prediction of human CL, the allometric equation has the following form:

$$CL = a \times W^b \qquad (4.2)$$

or

$$\log(CL) = \log(a) + b \times \log(W) \left[linearized\ form\ of\ equation \right]$$

Fig. 4.2 Representative plot showing simple allometry for *CL*

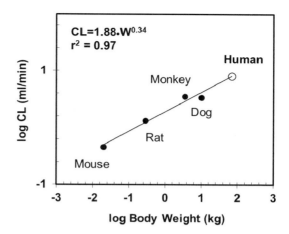

For the prediction of human *CL*, the a and b are estimated by performing linear regression on a plot of log *CL* versus log body weight consisting of *CL* estimates from preclinical species (Fig. 4.2). Predicted human *CL* is extrapolated from the regression line. Allometry assumes that *CL* is a function of body weight. It is of limited value for drugs where there are species specific differences in drug metabolism, plasma protein binding, of if different clearance mechanisms are operational across species.

4.2.3   The Rule of Exponents

A common correction that is made to simple allometry predictions of clearance is termed the "Rule of Exponents". The correction method involves using maximum life potential (*MLP*) or Brain Weight (*BrW*) to correct the simple allometric equation. The determination of which correction to use is based on the value of the allometric exponent (*b*) from the simple allometry plot.

b <0.7 use simple allometry.
0.7 ≤*b* <1.0 Use *MLP* Correction
b ≥1.0 use *BrW* correction.

The *MLP* correction and the *BrW* correction involves the following alterations to the simple allometric equation:

Maximum life span (*MLP*) correction:

$$CL \times MLP = a \times W^b \tag{4.3}$$

Brain weight (*BrW*) correction:

$$CL \times BrW = a \times W^b \qquad (4.4)$$

4.2.4   Other Human CL Prediction Methods Based on Allometric Principles

Other means of human clearance prediction based on allometry or allometric principles include:

4.2.5   Two Species Allometry

This method utilizes *in vivo* data from only two preclinical species (Tang et al. 2007).

$$CL_{human} = a_{rat-dog} \times W^{0.628} \qquad (4.5)$$

$$CL_{human} = a_{rat-monkey} \times W^{0.650} \qquad (4.6)$$

4.2.5.1   Allometry with Unbound Clearance (CL_u)

This method is similar to simple allometry but uses CL_u rather than *CL*.

$$CL_u = a \times W^b \qquad (4.7)$$

$CL_u = CL/f_u$; f_u = fraction unbound in plasma.

4.2.5.2   Tang and Mayersohn (2005)

A method that enhances the predictivity of allometry, in particular in case of "vertical allometry". Standard allometry is performed to determine the value of "*a*" (=coefficient of allometric equation) and the human clearance is obtained using the following equation:

$$CL = 33.35 \times \left(a / Rf_u \right)^{0.77} \qquad (4.8)$$

a = coefficient of standard allometric equation; $Rf_u = f_{u,rat}/f_{u,human}$.

4.2.6 Single Species Scaling

Single species scaling is based on direct extrapolation of the clearance in a particular preclinical species using a fixed exponent (usually 0.75) and with or without protein binding correction. In the latter case the equation is:

$$Cl_{u,human} = Cl_{u,animal} \times \left(W_{human} / W_{animal} \right)^{0.75} \tag{4.9}$$

4.2.7 Single Species Liver Blood Flow Method

The single species blood flow method uses the clearance as percentage of liver blood flow in preclinical species as predictor of human clearance as shown in the equation below. Ward and Smith (2004) suggested that the monkey is most predictive. This method of *CL* prediction based on in vivo data that does not rely on allometry.

$$CL_{human} = CL_{animal} \times \left(Q_{human} / Q_{animal} \right) \tag{4.10}$$

4.2.8 Simple Allometry for Prediction of Human V_d

Similar to *CL*, the allometric equation for the volume of distribution has the following form:

$$V_d = a \times W^b \text{ or}$$
$$\log(V_d) = \log(a) + b \times \log(W) \left[\text{linearized form of equation}\right] \tag{4.11}$$

Simple allometry has been used to predict volume of distribution with reasonable degree of success. Corrections to simple allometry such as the "Rule of Exponents" are not applied to predictions of V_d. A representative plot of simple allometry for volume of distribution prediction is shown in Fig. 4.3.

4.2.9 Other Human V_d Prediction Methods Based on Allometric Principles

4.2.9.1 Allometry with Unbound Clearance ($V_{d\,u}$)

This method is similar to simple allometry but uses $V_{d\,u}$ rather than V_d.

Fig. 4.3 Representative plot showing simple allometry for V_d

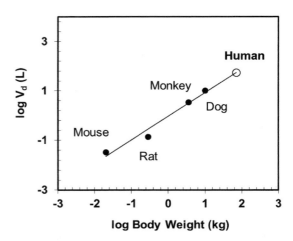

$$V_{d,u} = a \times W^b \qquad (4.12)$$

$V_{d,u} = V_d/f_u$; f_u = fraction unbound in plasma.

4.2.10 Single Species Scaling

Single species scaling is based on the similarity in V_d across species. Some have advocated an identical body weight normalized V_d in humans as in preclinical species, but it is more common to apply a correction factor for differences in plasma protein binding.

$$V_{d,u,human} = V_{d,u,animal} \times \left(f_{u,human} / f_{u,animal} \right) \qquad (4.13)$$

Opinions are divided about the most predictive preclinical animal model for humans. Hosea et al. (2009) observed good prediction of human pharmacokinetics using only rat data, which is also more practical than obtaining dog and/or monkey data. Other single species scaling methods were proposed by Tang et al. (2007).

4.2.11 Human PK Prediction Based on *In Vitro* Studies

Methods of predicting human pharmacokinetics relying on *in vitro* studies rely on in vitro to in vivo extrapolation which is the process by which *in vitro* data is scaled to the *in vivo* situation. Most human PK predictions using *in vitro* data focus on prediction of human CL with an emphasis on hepatic CL ($CL_{hepatic}$) as the liver is the primary organ of elimination for most small molecules. This section will focus on

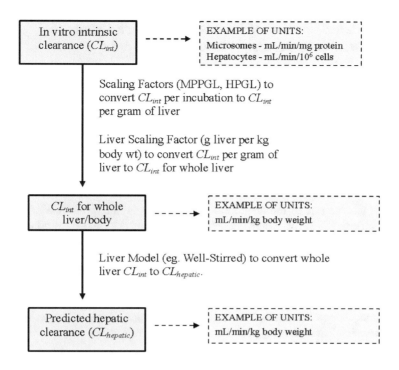

MPPGL – microsomal protein per gram of liver
HPGL – hepatocytes per gram of liver

Fig. 4.4 Flowchart depicting the process of *In Vitro-In Vivo* extrapolation

the liver as the organ of interest. A flowchart of the process of *in vitro* to *in vivo* extrapolation is shown below (Fig. 4.4).

As mentioned above, in this chapter, we will only be covering hepatic clearance. For drugs/ compounds that are eliminated *via* organs other than the liver, estimated organ clearances can be summed together get an estimate of total body clearance.

4.2.12   In Vitro Methods of Determining Intrinsic Clearance

Metabolic intrinsic clearance is a measure of the ability of hepatocytes to eliminate drug/ compound irrespective of other external factors such as protein binding and hepatic blood flow. Determination of metabolic intrinsic clearance can be accomplished using traditional enzyme kinetics methodologies or using substrate depletion methods.

4.2.13 Determination of Intrinsic Clearance Using Michaelis-Menten Kinetic Parameters

The relationship between the rate of a metabolic reaction and the substrate concentration is depicted in the Fig. 4.5 below:

The Michaelis-Menten equation describes this relationship for many metabolic reactions. The Michaelis-Menten equation is as follows:

$$v = \frac{V_{max} \times C}{K_m + C} \qquad (4.14)$$

where v is the rate of the metabolic reaction; V_{max} is maximum rate of the metabolic reaction; K_m is the Michaelis-Menten constant (i.e. substrate concentration where v is ½ of V_{max}); C is concentration of the substrate (i.e. drug/ compound of interest)

Michaelis-Menten kinetic parameters can be determined using in vitro under conditions of linearity with respect to incubation time and either microsomal protein concentrations (for microsomal incubations) or number of cells (for hepatocyte incubations). Once Michaelis-Menten kinetic parameters are estimated, the metabolic intrinsic clearance (CL_{int}) can be calculated as follows:

$$CL_{int} = \frac{V_{max}}{K_m + C} \qquad (4.15)$$

or $\qquad CL_{int} = \dfrac{V_{max}}{K_m}$ under linear conditions where $C \ll K_m$.

Based upon the above equations, CL_{int} is concentration dependent at high substrate concentrations approaching K_m. For most drugs, the concentrations administered in vivo are under conditions of linearity with respect to CL_{int}. CL_{int} estimated from in vitro incubations are in units of vol/time/mg of microsomal protein for microsomes (eg. µL/min/mg microsomal protein) and vol/time/number of cells for hepatocytes (eg. µL/min/10^6 cells).

Fig. 4.5 Plot of relationship between metabolic reaction rate (v) and substrate concentration (C)

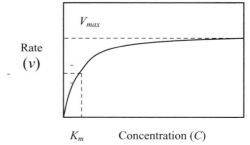

Determination of CL_{int} from Michaelis-Menten kinetic parameters can be labour intensive. As can be deduced from Fig. 4.5 in vitro incubations must be performed at multiple substrate concentrations for a good estimate of V_{max} and K_m. In addition, the metabolite reaction that is being monitored must be the formation of a major metabolite for a primary metabolic pathway for a prediction to be accurate. Alternatively, in a case where there is multiple major metabolic pathways responsible for drug elimination, the formation rates of the primary metabolites from these multiple pathways must be monitored, CL_{int} of each pathway must be estimated and summed together to get the overall CL_{int}. Substrate depletion rate may also be estimated at a range of substrate concentrations to estimate a hybrid overall apparent V_{max} and K_m. Regardless, every method utilizing Michaelis-Menten kinetic parameters requires that incubations must be performed at a wide range of substrate concentrations. Due to the more resource intensive nature of this method of intrinsic clearance estimation, substrate depletion estimation methods performed at one substrate concentrations where $C << K_m$ have become common.

4.2.14 Determination of Intrinsic Clearance Using Substrate Depletion Method at a Single Substrate Concentration (In Vitro $t_{1/2}$ Method)

Metabolic Intrinsic Clearance can be estimated using the *in vitro* half-life of a microsome or hepatocyte incubation. Using this method, the substrate concentration must be less than K_m (commonly 1 µM). The following equation is used to estimate the CL_{int} from the in vitro $t_{1/2}$.

$$CL_{int} = \frac{0.693}{t_{1/2(in\ vitro)}} \times \frac{V_{incubation}}{P_{microsome}} \tag{4.16}$$

where $t_{1/2(in\ vitro)}$ is the in vitro half-life; $V_{incubation}$ is the volume of the incubation; $P_{microsome}$ is the amount of microsomal protein in the incubation

If $t_{1/2(in\ vitro)}$ is in minutes, $V_{incubation}$ is in µL and $P_{microsome}$ is in mg than CL_{int} will be in units of µL/min/mg microsomal protein. It is important to keep track of units when performing in vitro-in vivo extrapolation.

The *in vitro* $t_{1/2}$ method can also be applied to hepatocytes where $P_{microsome}$ would be replaced with "the number of hepatocytes in the incubation". Since the number of hepatocytes in an incubation is usually expressed as "X $\times 10^6$ cells", the units for CL_{int}, in the preceding example, would be µL/min/10^6 cells.

4.2.15   Scaling Factors for In Vitro-In Vivo Extrapolation

In this section we present scaling factors for the conversion of CL_{int} estimated from in vitro incubations to CL_{int} for the whole liver or body (Table 4.1).

For monkeys, it is recommended to use the values for humans as a detailed analysis of MPPGL and HPGL is not available currently (Table 4.2).

4.2.16   Liver Models for Estimation of Hepatic Clearance

Conversion of CL_{int} for the whole liver/body to hepatic clearance which includes the impact of physiological factors such as blood flow and protein binding involves the use of a liver model such as the well-stirred model, the parallel tube model, or dispersion model. None of the models have been shown to be superior to the others (Baranczewski et al. 2006) so for simplicity the equation for the well-stirred model is presented below.

$$CL_{hepatic} = Q \frac{f_u CL_{int}}{f_u CL_{int} + Q} \tag{4.17}$$

where $CL_{hepatic}$ is the hepatic clearance; f_u is the unbound fraction; Q is the hepatic blood flow.

Table 4.1 Liver microsome and hepatocyte scaling factors for various species

	Human	Rat	Dog
MPPGL (mg microsomal protein per gram liver)	32 (95% CI: 29 to 34)	61 (95% CI: 47 to 75)	55 (95% CI: 48 to 62)
HPGL (×10⁶ hepatocytes per gram of liver)	99 (95% CI: 74 to 131)	163 (95% CI: 127 to 199)	169 (95% CI: 131 to 207)

CI confidence interval
Adapted from Smith et al. 2008 and Barter et al. 2007

Table 4.2 Liver weight and liver scaling factor (g liver per kg body weight) for various species

	Mouse (0.02 kg)	Rat (0.25 kg)	Dog (10 kg)	Monkey (5 kg)	Human (70 kg)
Species (weight)					
Liver weight (g)	1.75 g	10.0 g	320 g	150 g	1800 g
Liver scaling factor (g liver per kg body weight)	87.5 g/kg	40 g/kg	32 g/kg	30 g/kg	25.7 g/kg

Adapted from Davies and Morris 1993

Values for hepatic blood flow are presented in Table 3.2.

In vitro – in vivo extrapolation is usually "validated" by determining if the *in vitro* ADME data correctly predict the clearance observed in preclinical studies. Although this is valuable, it is possible that human clearance involves pathways distinctly different from preclinical species, which renders this "validation" of limited value.

Use of the well-stirred model for basic and neutral drugs/compounds often does not require the inclusion of microsomal protein binding f_u in the calculation. Often for basic and neutral drugs/compounds, f_u often cancels out with f_{umic} (unbound fraction in microsomes) (Obach 1999). The well-stirred model equation including f_{umic} is as follows:

$$CL_{hepatic} = Q \frac{f_u \dfrac{CL_{int}}{f_{umic}}}{f_u \dfrac{CL_{int}}{f_{umic}} + Q} \tag{4.18}$$

In contrast to plasma protein binding, microsomal binding, f_{umic}, is generally not species dependent provided the microsomal protein concentration is the same (Zhang et al. 2010).

4.2.17 Oie-Tozer Method for Prediction of Volume of Distribution

In the Oie-Tozer method the unbound fraction in human plasma and the average unbound fraction in tissues from preclinical species (assumed to be equal to the unbound fraction in human tissues), combined with appropriate human values for plasma and fluid volumes, are used to predict the human volume of distribution (Obach et al. 1997).

$$V_{d,human} = V_p + \left(f_{u,human} \times V_e \right) + \left[\left(1 - f_{u,human} \right) \times \left(\frac{R_e}{i} \right) \times V_p \right] + \left(V_r \times \frac{f_{u,human}}{f_{ut,species\,average}} \right) \tag{4.19}$$

V_p plasma volume; V_e extracellular fluid volume; V_r "remainder of the fluid volume; R_e/i ratio of binding proteins in extracellular fluid (except plasma) to binding proteins in plasma; $f_{ut,species\,average}$ average unbound fraction in tissues from preclinical species.

4.2.18 Prediction of Human Fraction Absorbed

The fraction absorbed is influenced by the intestinal solubility of the drug and the permeability across enterocytes. Solubility and dissolution rate studies can predict if absorption is limited by the solubility of the drug, and this is reflected by the maximum absorbable dose. Note that the magnitude of the anticipated human dose should be taken into consideration as well. *In vitro* permeability studies involving Caco-2 or MDCK cells or PAMPA provide a good idea about the intrinsic permeability of the drug. Details are provided in Sect. 6.2.5. Efflux by transporters can limit the fraction absorbed, but intestinal transporters can be saturated relatively easy. Finally, preclinical PK data can be used to predict F_a and the first-order absorption rate constant (k_a). The fraction absorbed combined with knowledge of intestinal metabolism and systemic clearance can be used to predict F.

Preclinical Models for Human Drug Absorption
Although monkeys may be good models to predict F_h in humans, $F_a \times F_g$ is frequently substantially smaller in monkeys than in humans for drugs that undergo a significant degree of metabolism (Akabane et al. 2010). This probably reflects an increased capacity for intestinal metabolism in monkeys, because an earlier study showed that F_a in monkeys correlates well with F_a in humans (Chiou and Buehler 2002).

Although dogs are commonly used to study oral absorption, F_a in dogs is frequently larger than F_a in humans (Chiou et al. 2000). In addition, t_{max} tends to be longer in humans than in dogs. The correlation between F_a in rats and humans is more robust (Chiou and Barve 1998).

4.2.19 Context of Confidence in Human PK Predictions

Predictions of human pharmacokinetics are performed extensively using preclinical information and serve to triage and select compounds under consideration for development. The confidence and value of the prediction is in large part determined by the input. At an earlier stage, the predictions are based on limited data sets (in vitro and rodent in vivo data) and the goal is usually to categorize compounds and identify compounds worth pursuing further in preclinical studies. Once a more complete data set is available, it is possible to make human PK predictions with a more complete understanding of a specific compound's in vivo behavior. Even at this stage, the predictions are more a reflection of assumed risk with compounds having favorable PK properties being less of a risk to advance. Indeed, the most successful clearance methods generally have a success rate of 60 to 80% within two-fold. Indeed, Beaumont and Smith (2009) commented that *"Generation of further large amount of preclinical information on a compound with uncertain human pharmacokinetic prediction tends to add confusion rather than clarity."*

4.3 Pharmacokinetic/ Modeling and Human Dose Prediction

Pharmacokinetic/pharmacodynamic (PK/PD) modeling serves to link anticipated human pharmacokinetics to a pharmacodynamic endpoint in order to provide a predicted pharmacologically active dose in humans (Fig. 4.6). These predicted "human doses" serves as an integrated assessment that incorporates all that is known about the pharmacokinetics and pharmacodynamics of a drug candidate. Similar to predictions of human pharmacokinetics, the predicted human pharmacologically active dose can serve as a measure of assumed risk with compounds have lower predicted doses being less risk to advance to development. Further, PK/PD modelling using preclinical data during the drug discovery phase can aid in the prediction of efficacious human doses and selection of dose regimens for clinical testing.

4.3.1 Pharmacodynamic Endpoint

As illustrated in Fig. 4.6, prediction of a pharmacologically active dose requires a pharmacodynamic endpoint that can be obtained from *in vitro* or *in vivo* sources. An appropriate pharmacodynamic endpoint can be as simple as maintaining a concentration (such as an IC_{50} or IC_{90} from an in vitro assay) for a specific period of time or achieving a drug exposure (i.e. C_{max} or AUC) that is associated with an acceptable level of activity in a preclinical efficacy model. The pharmacodynamic endpoint should be selected based on where anticipated activity is expected to be observed in the patient population. In its simplest form, PK/PD modeling involves using predicted human pharmacokinetics (as described in Sect. 4.2) to construct a PK model in order to identify doses that meet the chosen concentration based pharmacodynamic endpoints (eg. IC_{50}, IC_{90}, C_{max}, AUC) described above.

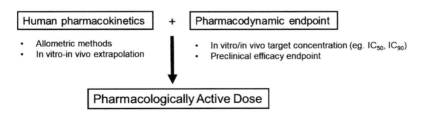

Fig. 4.6 Process of prediction of pharmacologically active dose in humans

Often for novel targets it is difficult to determine what is considered an appropriate pharmacodynamic endpoint to target for predicting active human doses. A common endpoint is coverage of an IC_{50} concentration (for a compound that is an inhibitor) for the entire dosing interval. An optimal target if a compound's tolerability will allow would be coverage of an IC_{90} concentration for the entire dosing interval. A compound that has the appropriate safety profile to continuously cover the "higher bar" IC_{90} concentration target will allow proper interrogation of the novel first-in class target in phase II "proof of concept" clinical trials.

4.3.2 Delayed Onset of Pharmacodynamic Effect and the Counter-Clockwise Hysteresis

Pharmacological responses can have delayed onset and lag behind plasma/ serum concentrations. Observations of a delayed onset of action may be due to factors such as:

1. Rate-limiting distribution of drug to tissue where the drug biological target resides (e.g. drugs that target the central nervous system can show slow distribution into brain tissue).
2. Indirect action of the drug on the pharmacological effect (i.e. drug acts on biological target that is upstream of the pharmacological effect which causes a temporal disconnect between drug concentration and effect).

Time lags between drug concentrations and pharmacological responses can be observed as counter-clockwise hysteresis in plots of pharmacological effect versus drug concentration (Fig. 4.7). The open circles in the effect versus concentration plot in Fig. 4.7 designate serial observations with the numbering (1–5) designating

Fig. 4.7 A counterclockwise hysteresis associated with a delayed onset of effect. The open circles (1 to 5) designated effect versus concentration for this phenomenon

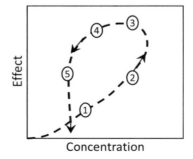

Concentration

the sequential order of each observation. Clockwise hysteresis can also occur but are less common. Drug tolerance is a phenomenon that can result in a clockwise hysteresis in plots of effect versus concentration. Finally, hysteresis can distort our understanding of concentration-effect relationships. In situations where they are observed, PK/PD modeling becomes a very important tool for characterization of concentration-effect relationships.

In situations where a compound shows a delayed onset of effect, the use of a more complex PK/PD modelling is more ideal. Biophase distribution model or indirect response models are two types of PK/PD models that can be used to characterize delayed onset of effects and predict active doses.

Alternate Means to Deal with Hysteresis

Hysteresis can distort concentration-effect relationships. As mentioned, biophase distribution models and indirect response models can characterize concentration-effect relationships despite the presence of hysteresis. An alternate means of dealing with hysteresis is through study design. Preclinical PK/PD studies can be performed using steady-state infusions to achieve a broad range of concentrations required to properly define the concentration-effect relationship. A steady-state infusion study design may allow for characterization of concentration-effect relationships without using more complex biophase distribution and indirect response models. However, this study design is typically more labor and resource intensive.

4.4 Physiologically-Based Pharmacokinetic Models

Physiologically-based pharmacokinetic models are more sophisticated and are built around a wide range of parameters that describe the normal physiology of the human or animal body. They are made up of multiple compartments, each representing a predefined tissue or connected via blood or lymph flow (Fig. 4.8).

Parameters that are included in the model are blood flow to organs, weight of organs, drug metabolizing enzymes in the liver and elsewhere in the body, drug transporters in the body, etc. Absorption is frequently modeled using the Advanced Compartmental and Transit (ACAT) model or the Advanced Dissolution, Absorption and Metabolism (ADAM) model. These models describe the various compartments of the intestinal tract in detail and include details about:

- rate constants for gastric emptying
- intestinal compartmental transit time
- local permeability of intestinal wall
- pH of each compartment
- volume and surface area of each compartment
- enterocytic blood flow

Fig. 4.8 Diagram of a whole body physiologically-based pharmacokinetic model

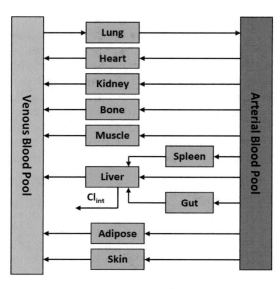

⟶ **Represents blood/lymph flows and clearances**

Table 4.3 Commercially available PBPK models

Software	Vendor
Cloe PK	Cyprotex
GastroPlus	Simulations plus
PK-Sim	Bayer
Simcyp	Certara

The model will determine the extent of dissolution, absorption and metabolism by enterocytes for each compartment. The input for the PBPK model are parameters that specifically describe the compound of interest: pKa, lipophilicity, solubility in various media, in vitro permeability, in vitro metabolic stability, CYP inhibition, etc. In addition, the dose, dosing route and dosing regimen is provided. Commercially available PBPK models are listed in Table 4.3.

The output of the PBPK model is a concentration – time profile. For some models it is possible to provide a population range instead of an average profile. PBPK models are quite powerful and they are extensively used for prediction of the following:

- Human and animal pharmacokinetics
- Food effect
- Formulation effect
- Dosing regimen effect
- Drug-drug interactions via competitive and time-dependent CYP inhibition and CYP induction (Simcyp)

The overall role that PBPK modeling can play in candidate translational characterization is that PBPK models can be applied to predict human pharmacokinetics for purposes of human dose/regimen prediction. In addition, these models can be used to perform an early assessment of the drug-drug interaction potential of a drug candidate.

4.5 Toxicokinetics and Safety Margins

Integration of the results of preclinical toxicology studies serves as one of the final exercises in the evaluation of promising drug candidates. The dosing of small molecule drug candidates is typically limited by toxicity making toxicokinetics of a compound and the associated predicted safety margins important to compound evaluation.

4.5.1 Toxicokinetics

Toxicokinetics (TK) refers to the application of pharmacokinetics to assess the relationship of compound exposure and toxicological effect in preclinical toxicology studies. The principle pharmacokinetic parameters used in toxicokinetics are:

- C_{max} – the highest concentration that is observed
- t_{max} – the time that C_{max} is observed
- AUC – area under the concentration time curve

These three parameters characterize the rate and extent of absorption. For multiple dose toxicology studies, these parameters are evaluated on the first and last day of dosing. The TK parameters evaluated on the last day of dosing are typically associated with the toxicological effect. Other parameters (such as $t_{1/2}$) may be reported but have less importance as often the doses used in toxicology studies are high and the pharmacokinetics are often nonlinear. For toxicology studies performed in rodents, small blood volume may require that a limited amount of blood samples be taken per animal. This leads to TK parameters being evaluated using a pooled plasma concentration-time profiles from all animals in a particular dose group.

4.5.2 Safety Margins

A predicted safety margin based on preclinical studies is one of the final assessments when performing a candidate translational characterization. The information used in the assessment of a preclinical safety margin is shown in Fig. 4.9 and represents much of the preclinical information gathered for a drug candidate.

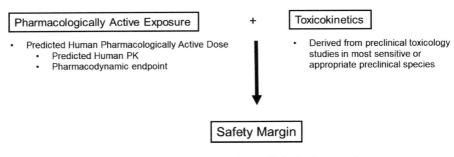

Fig. 4.9 Information required in the assessment of a preclinical safety margin

The preclinical safety margin is estimated using the exposure (typically C_{max} and AUC at steady-state for multiple dose toxicology studies) from what would be considered a "safe" or acceptable dose in the most sensitive or appropriate preclinical species. The exposure is divided by the corresponding predicted pharmacologically active exposure in humans. Safety margins for both C_{max} and AUC can be evaluated. A higher preclinical safety margin represents a more favorable drug candidate. The safety margins are usually greater than 20 for a non-oncology indication while a value of 2 can argue for a clinical testing of an oncology drug candidate. For an entity such as antibody-drug conjugate where the dosed form is not directly responsible for toxicities, a safety margin can also be represented by doses instead of exposures.

References

Akabane T, Tabata K, Kadono K et al (2010) A comparison of pharmacokinetics between humans and monkeys. Drug Metab Dispos 38:308–316

Baranczewski P, Stanczak A, Sundberg K et al (2006) Introduction to *in vitro* estimation of metabolic stability and drug interactions of new chemical entities in drug discovery and development. Pharmacol Rep 58:453–472

Barter ZE, Bayliss MK, Beaune PH et al (2007) Scaling factors for the extrapolation of *in vivo* metabolic drug clearance from *in vitro* data: reaching a consensus on values of human microsomal protein and hepatocellularity per gram of liver. Curr Drug Metab 8:33–45

Beaumont K, Smith DA (2009) Does human pharmacokinetic prediction add significant value to compound selection in drug discovery research? Curr Opin Drug Disc Dev 12:61–71

Chiou WL, Barve A (1998) Linear correlation of the fraction of oral dose absorbed of 64 drugs between humans and rats. Pharm Res 15:1792–1795

Chiou WL, Jeong HY, Chung SM et al (2000) Evaluation of using dog as an animal model to study the fraction of oral dose absorbed of 43 drugs in humans. Pharm Res 17:135–140

Chiou WL, Buehler PW (2002) Comparison of oral absorption and bioavailability of drugs between monkey and human. Pharm Res 19:868–874

Davies B, Morris T (1993) Physiological parameters in laboratory animals and humans. Pharm Res 10:1093–1095

Hosea N, Collard WT, Cole S et al (2009) Prediction of human pharmacokinetics from preclinical information: comparative accuracy of quantitative prediction approaches. J Clin Pharmacol 49:513–533

Kola I, Landis J (2004) Can the pharmaceutical industry reduce attrition rates? Nat Rev Drug Disc 3:711–716

Obach RS, Baxter JG, Liston TE et al (1997) The prediction of human pharmacokinetic parameters from preclinical and *in vitro* metabolism data. J Pharmacol Exp Ther 283:46–58

Obach RS (1999) Prediction of human clearance of twenty-nine drugs from hepatic microsomal intrinsic clearance data: an examination of *in vitro* half-life approach and nonspecific binding to microsomes. Drug Metab Dispos 27:1350–1359

Smith R, Jones RD, Ballard PG et al (2008) Determination of microsome and hepatocyte scaling factors for *in vitro*/*in vivo* extrapolation in the rat and dog. Xenobiotica 38:1386–1398

Tang H, Mayersohn M (2005) A novel method for prediction of human drug clearance by allometric scaling. Drug Metab Dispos 33:1297–1303

Tang H, Hussain A, Leal M et al (2007) Interspecies prediction of human drug clearance based on scaling data from one or two animal species. Drug Metab Dispos 35:1886–1893

Ward KW, Smith BR (2004) A comprehensive quantitative and qualitative evaluation of extrapolation of intravenous pharmacokinetic parameters from rat, dog, and monkey to humans. I Clearance Drug Metab Dispos 32:603–611

Zhang Y, Yao L, Lin J et al (2010) Lack of appreciable species differences in nonspecific microsomal binding. J Pharm Sci 99:3620–3627

Chapter 5
Q&A of DMPK Issues and Tools for Drug Discovery

Contents

Abstract This section addresses some typical DMPK questions that an ADME scientist encounters during drug discovery support. These questions are addressed by means of general concepts, experimental approaches, and examples. They are also linked to other sections for the ease of search and understanding.

Keywords Strategy · Pharmacokinetics · Drug metabolism · Drug transport · Drug discovery · Drug development

© Springer Nature Switzerland AG 2022
S. C. Khojasteh et al., *Discovery DMPK Quick Guide*,
https://doi.org/10.1007/978-3-031-10691-0_5

Abbreviations

BCRP   Breast cancer resistance protein (ABCG2)
MATE   Multidrug and toxin extrusion transporters (SLC47As)
OAT   Organic anion transporters (SCL22A family)
OATP   Organic anion transporting polypeptides (SLCO family)
OCT   Organic cation transporters (SCL22A family)
P-gp   P-glycoprotein (ABCB1)

5.1   ADME Discovery Strategy

5.1.1   What Is the Minimum Set of In Vitro Assays Needed During the Drug Discovery Process?

The minimum set of ADME assays depends on the molecule that is being optimized and the ADME challenges encountered by previous molecules. Also, if a project is further along in the drug discovery process, it is customary for more assays to be incorporated in the screening cascade and the assays themselves are more detailed as well. Generally, the assays should be picked based on the molecular properties, site of action, and stage in discovery (Sect. 6.1). Two things are critical in the discovery stages when it comes to ADME assays:

1. the relevance of the output of the assay. The relevant assay needs to be viewed based on the behavior and characteristics of the molecule. This is called a 'fit for purpose' approach. For example, liver microsome stability is not an appropriate assay to use with peptides since many cytosolic hydrolases are not present in this matrix. The assay will not give accurate results for these compounds since the relevant enzymes are not present.
2. the cycle time between design, data generation, assessment, and a new design. Shorter cycles in generating data allow for more designs to be made and cycle times are more important in an increasingly competitive environment with many companies working on the same target. Data quality also plays an important role in determining timelines. If quantitative structural activity relationship (QSAR) models are available, then in vitro assays may be used as confirmation and for spot checking.

Based on the stage of the project, more properties can be assessed to understand potential liabilities. If a critical liability is identified, then it makes sense to move the assay for assessing this particular liability earlier in the screening cascade. As a project progresses, the quantity of data increases for proper assessment of the potential to proceed to development with that molecule and to differentiate it from close-in analogs. Here are a set of assays that provide valuable information in early drug discovery (O'Brien and Moghaddam 2015):

- Calculated physicochemical properties: logP, pKa, TPSA, hydrogen bond donor/acceptor (HBD/HBA)
- Kinetic solubility measurements: This result has a high impact on all other measurements as a poorly soluble compound may result in an unreliable read out from many assays (in vitro potency, selectivity, ADME, etc.).
- In vitro ADME properties: chemical stability, enzymatic stability (e.g. liver microsomes, hepatocytes, plasma), permeability, plasma protein binding, CYP inhibition/induction (Chap. 6). As mentioned, QSAR models for ADME properties (metabolic stability, permeability, others) can play an important role in bypassing some of the studies in the laboratory. In silico calculations also allow doing virtual analysis prior to compound synthesis.

5.1.2 Should Plasma Protein Binding (PPB) Be Optimized to Improve PK?

The short answer is no, as described in Sect. 3.6. Plasma protein binding remains a complex issue and is misinterpreted by many. Indeed, many argue that plasma protein binding needs to be 'optimized' and that high plasma protein binding is an undesirable property. However, there are many successful drugs with high plasma protein binding. With some exceptions as highlighted in Sect. 3.6, the goal of the drug discovery effort should be on optimizing the amount of **unbound** (also called 'free') drug per mg of drug administered, because it is the **unbound** drug that can interact with the therapeutic target. In addition, drugs are metabolized based on the **unbound** drug level available to interact with the drug metabolizing enzymes. Thus, it is the unbound intrinsic clearance that should be reduced, as this will result in a lower efficacious dose. (Of course, improving the potency is an alternative path towards a lower dose.) A high degree of plasma protein binding will increase the total (bound + unbound) drug levels, but plasma protein binding will not affect the unbound drug levels and, therefore, high plasma protein binding will not negatively affect the efficacious dose (again with some exceptions as highlighted in Sect. 3.6). Finally, plasma protein binding is a function of lipophilicity and increases with increasing logP while solubility generally decreases with increasing logP. The unbound clearance and unbound volume of distribution also increase with lipophilicity. Moreover, the effects on both clearance and volume of distribution almost cancel each other out and the half life may stay roughly the same or may slightly increase with increasing logP. In the end, it is this deep understanding of the impact of various physicochemical parameters on ADME parameters, such as absorption and clearance, that is essential in drug discovery. These physicochemical parameters may influence plasma protein binding, but plasma protein binding does not need to be 'optimized'. See Sect. 3.6 for details.

5.1.3   Can Drug Delivery Systems Save a Challenging ADME Drug?

The main objective of drug formulation is to enhance the bioavailability (exposure) of drugs (Singh et al. 2020) if the bioavailability is low due to poor intrinsic solubility or dissolution. Drug delivery systems are considered in two broad categories: (1) formulations and (2) devices. In each case, it can enable a drug to reach the site of action. Drug delivery systems have advanced in recent years, which allows more-challenging candidates to enter development. This has created new opportunities for addressing certain kinds of ADME shortcomings, such as poor absorption, lack of tissue uptake, and a short half-life.

Examples are (Narang and Mahato 2010):

• Lipid-based drug delivery systems using lipid excipients or surfactants/co-solvents have beene deployed to enhance solubility and absorption, resulting in higher bioavailability in the gastrointestinal tract.
• Molecular carrier systems (e.g. cyclodextrin-encapsulated drugs) to modulate local toxicity in the GI tract and prevent the drug from crashing out in the intestine.
• Nanoparticles have been extensively used to increase solubility and bioavailability, reduce toxicities, and enhance controlled release (Zhang et al. 2013). In addition, nanoparticles can be surface-functionalized with a variety of ligands to enhance circulation half-life and uptake in (specific) tissues.

5.1.4   How to Select Toxicity Species at the Drug Discovery Stage?

The guidance around toxicity species selection revolves around two concepts:

(a) Pharmacologically relevant species (out of scope of this book).
(b) Metabolite generation and exposure.

First, assays need to be developed to determine the in vitro potency of the drug in – most commonly – mouse, rat, dog and cynomolgous monkey relative to human. Pronounced species differences can guide species selection for toxicity studies to ensure that on-target toxicity is reliably evaluated in preclinical tolerability studies. Second, metabolic profiles generated in hepatocytes or liver microsomes are used to determine species similarity or differences in exposure to various metabolites (Table 6.S.2). The side-by-side comparison of the type and quantity of metabolites in various species is used for species selection (Sect. 6.2.5). One of the common ways in this comparison is normalizing the MS response across the species for each metabolite. This allows for determining the major primary metabolites formed and hence selection of tox species based on metabolites formed in comparison to humans.

A few considerations:

- The in vitro formation of metabolites does not guarantee that any of the metabolites circulate. Currently, there are no practical predictive models or assays that can be used to estimate the metabolites that circulate. However, attempts have been made to model the circulating metabolites of midazolam, and it is complicated requiring a lot of data for both the parent compound and the various metabolites (Nguyen et al. 2016).
- Preclinical circulating metabolites can be identified from discovery PK or TK studies as part of metabolite identification from in vivo samples. Although circulating metabolites in preclinical species may not be as prominent as circulating metabolites in humans, it is useful to know if there are any circulating metabolites in tox species. Moreover, the exposure of the parent drug achieved in toxicity studies is usually far greater than in human studies and, therefore, sufficient coverage may be achieved for metabolites that are – relative to the parent compound – less abundant in preclinical species.

See also Sect. 5.2.2.

5.1.5   What Are the ADME Challenges to Be Considered with New Modalities?

New modalities are captured in Sects. 2.1 and 2.4. Different technologies are deployed for optimizing these types of molecules. Many of them need to be able to address both potency and ADME properties at this time. Based on specific liabilities of these new modalities, the assay focus will be different. For example, macrocyclic peptides suffer from poor permeability, and bifunctional degraders suffer from poor solubility (Cantrill et al. 2020). Many new chromatographic-based measurements have been developed for measuring physicochemical properties. These assays, such as ePSA (Goetz et al. 2014) and IAM, are compatible with using trace amounts of material (see Sect. 6.2.5).

Relatively poor pharmacokinetic properties are often observed for new modalities. Note that these molecules may display asymmetry in terms of drug concentration in tissue versus plasma (Zhang et al. 2019). This difference means that plasma may be a poor predictor of tissue and, hence, efficacy.

5.2   Metabolism-Related Concerns

5.2.1   How to Determine the Safety Contribution of Metabolites?

See Sect. 5.1.4.

5.2.2   Is the Presence of Circulating Metabolites a Concern in Preclinical Species?

It is not unusual to detect abundant circulating metabolites in preclinical species. This information by itself does not point to any risk or liability for the compound. Indeed, the goal is not to optimize drugs for preclinical species - it is exposure in humans that matters. However, the observation may lead to additional investigations.

Note: (1) Observing a circulating metabolite in preclinical species does not necessarily indicate that the same metabolite will be found circulating in human. (2) Predicting circulating metabolites from in vitro metabolism assays in different species remains challenging.

ADME Consideration of a Circulating Metabolite:

- Bioanalytical concern: Can this metabolite interfere with detection of the parent drug? In many cases, conjugated metabolites such as glucuronides can fragment in the source of the mass spectrometer and, provided that they co-elute with the parent drug, result in over-estimation of the presence of the parent compound in circulation. Once this is known, chromatographic separation is essential to separate the analytes for more accurate measurement of the parent compound.
- Estimation of the amount of the metabolite: Mass spectrometry has revolutionized the detection of metabolites due to its very high sensitivity and selectivity. At the same time, without authentic standards, MS detection is an unreliable method for accurate quantitation of metabolites. The parent and its metabolites often have very different response factors due to their different ionization efficiencies. There are some methods describing normalization of ionization using nanospray (Hop et al. 2005; Hop 2006; Schadt et al. 2011), but this is not what is routinely used. A mixed-matrix method has been developed to qualify metabolite abundance in plasma across species (Takahashi et al. 2017). This method showed similar results to those obtained from validated bioanalytical methods. We think that this method, if done appropriately, has the opportunity to be considered by regulatory agencies for assessing relative exposure of metabolites between humans and animal species used in toxicology studies.
- The metabolite formed in the liver is often too polar to be permeable, and it, therefore, relies on drug transport to find its way into circulation. Many glucuronides may fall into this category. A high amount of circulating metabolite may be observed and this may be made worse by a very low volume of distribution of that metabolite. This particular observation means that the total amount of metabolite in the body would be limited, even though the quantity of the circulating metabolite may suggest otherwise. For this type of metabolite, it is very difficult to predict the circulating metabolite just based on the in vitro rate of formation. Metabolites may also have a lower clearance and, hence, longer half-life than the parent compound, which could result in accumulation of the metabolite in circulation. Is the circulating metabolite expected to be formed based on

hepatic metabolism? Based on the structure of the metabolite, one could consider what changes to make in the parent molecule to decrease clearance by removing the metabolic soft spot.

• Based on available data, is this metabolite formed in human? A metabolite may be formed in all species in vitro, however, in vitro and even preclinical in vivo studies have limitations in the prediction of metabolite circulation in humans because the expression of drug metabolizing enzymes can be very different between species. For example, the sulfonated metabolite of O-demethyl apixaban was a major circulating metabolite in humans, although only a low level of this metabolite was detected in preclinical species (Wang et al. 2009).

Pharmacological and toxicological questions that need to be asked about circulating metabolites:

1. Is the metabolite considered pharmacologically active (on target)? If active, how much is the metabolite's contribution to the total efficacy?
2. Does the metabolite have drug-like properties? For metabolites that do have drug-like properties and pharmacological activity, one must make sure that there is intellectual property protection. A case in point is terfenadine that gets metabolized to fexofenadine. Ultimately, the metabolite fexofenadine was developed into a successful drug without the hERG liability exhibited by terfenadine.
3. Is there a safety signal that could be attributed to circulating metabolites? This question basically asks if the metabolite could have off-target activity perhaps different than the parent compound. It is common for teams to think that metabolites contribute to or are responsible for the observed toxicity, but it is usually very difficult to find the true culprit and dissect the toxic properties of parent compounds and their metabolites in a timely fashion.

5.2.3   When to Perform Reaction Phenotyping?

Reaction phenotyping is used to determine the drug metabolizing enzyme(s) involved in the formation of a specific metabolite (method shared in Sect. 6.2.2). Typically, in-depth reaction phenotyping studies are performed later in the drug discovery process prior to candidate nomination or in early development. However, performing these types of studies to spot check chemical series enables understanding of a potential liability, such as significant metabolism by a polymorphic enzyme.

Polymorphic Enzymes

CYP: CYP1A2, CYP2C9, 2C19, 2D6 and 3A5 can have marked clinical impacts on their substrates (see Cases 2.10 and 3.3, and Sect. 3.4).

UGT: UGT1A1, 1A6, 1A7, 2B4, and UGT2B7 (Miners et al. 2002).

5.2.4 What Are the Challenges for Drugs for Which Glucuronidation or Aldehyde Oxidase Oxidation is the Major Route of Clearance?

Glucuronidation: UGT (Sect. 3.4)
- *In vitro* metabolism systems frequently underestimate *in vivo* glucuronidation metabolic clearance.
- Determine if the metabolism is mediated by a polymorphic enzyme (Sect. 5.2.3).
- UGT1A1 inhibitors (like atazanavir) could lead to bilirubinemia as bilirubin is metabolized through this pathway (Hahn et al. 2006).
- Selected glucuronides are inactivators of CYPs. For example, the glucuronide metabolites of gemfibrozil and clopidogrel are time-dependent inhibitors of CYP2C8 (Ma et al. 2017).
- Glucuronides, if excreted into the bile, can be deconjugated in the intestine and subsequently reabsorbed, i.e. enterohepatic recirculation.

Aldehyde Oxidase: AO (Sect. 3.4.1.2)
- *In vitro* metabolism systems could underestimate *in vivo* clearance.
- Dogs do not express active AO and therefore should not be used as a toxicological species, if this is an expected metabolic pathway in humans. If you include dogs in allometric scaling of a drug with a high AO clearance component, it may result in under-estimation of human clearance.
- Low solubility of AO metabolites is reported to cause kidney toxicity (Case 3.7).
- Mass spectral analysis may underestimate the extent of metabolite formation due to potential poor ionization effiency of lactams compared to heterocynm cles.

5.2.5 What to Do When a Compound Is Stable in **In Vitro** Metabolic Systems, but Has High Clearance **In Vivo**?

- If stable in liver microsomes: Liver microsomes plus NADPH cofactor targets only specific types of reactions, such as CYP and Flavin-containing monooxygenase (FMO). Systems like hepatocytes target a broader range of hepatic enzymes.
- The drug may be cleared unchanged and does not rely on metabolic pathways for elimination. Transporters could be involved.
- Saturation of drug metabolizing enzymes in the *in vitro* assays. Many times we assume $K_m >> 1$ µM. Therefore, lower concentrations need to be used.
- *In vitro* systems often underestimate clearance for most enzymes and this could be worse for glucuronidation or hydrolysis metabolism. If binding corrections are incorporated, better correlations usually are obtained.

5.2.6   How to Determine the Contribution of Metabolism (CL_m) to the Total In Vivo Clearance Pathways?

Determining the contribution of metabolism to the total clearance is not a trivial matter, especially at the early discovery stage. The BDDCS and ECCS (Sect. 2.1.2) can be used as guidance. These classification systems state that a permeable compound usually is cleared metabolically, otherwise it would need drug transport. These classification systems are considered a framework and are not quantitative. These methods do not offer information about the type of metabolic reaction and the rate. In our experience, the contribution of metabolism to the total clearance does not dramatically change from one species to another.

A metabolically stable compound in vitro could show extensive metabolism in vivo due to, for example, reabsorption-metabolism cycles (Zhang et al. 2021). Indeed, it is important not to mix up the rate and extent of metabolism. For example, vismodegib is extensively metabolized, but the rate is very slow and, hence, the half-life is long.

Here are some helpful type of studies:

- Consider using 1-aminobenzotriazole (ABT) to determine the cytochrome (CYP) contribution to the total clearance (*CL*). Note that with ABT, chronic studies can be performed because it is tolerated in rats (see Case 3.5).
- Review the *in vitro* (extrapolated from hepatocyte or liver microsomal intrinsic clearance) to *in vivo* correlation (IVIVC).
- Conduct bile-duct cannulation studies and collect urine to determine the biliary and renal clearance.
- If dose recovery is good, the percent of metabolites recovered represents the metabolic contribution to total clearance.

5.3   Drug Transporter-Related Concerns

Typically, an extensive assessment of drug transporters is not conducted during drug discovery which is the focus of this book, but rather it is part of drug development.

5.3.1   What Drug Transporters Could Be Subject to Drug-Drug Interaction?

Drug transporters are often considered from the perspectives of understanding PK properties and drug-drug interaction potential.

- Inhibition of transporters (P-gp, BCRP, OATP1B1/3, OAT1/3, OCT1/2, MATEs) can be a concern. Examples of clinically relevant transporter-based DDIs include the interactions between digoxin and quinidine, fexofenadine and ketoconazole, cimetidine and metformin, rosuvastatin and cyclosporine (Fromm et al. 1999; Simonson et al. 2004; Muller et al. 2018; Billington et al. 2019). The most pronounced drug-drug interactions are observed when the perpetrator drug inhibits multiple transporter pathways required for the clearance of a victim drug. In addition, the magnitude of transporter- mediated drug-drug intercation is usually much smaller than CYP-mediated drug-drug interaction.

• If intact excretion of the parent compound is a prominent clearance pathway, identification of the compound as a substrate would be important for the various transport scenarios described below.

Nine clinically important transporters are recommended in FDA DDI guidance for routine evaluation of DDI potential for drug candidates.

• efflux transporters: P-gp, BCRP, MATE1 and MATE2-K
• uptake transporters: OATP1B1, OATP1B3, OAT1, OAT3, and OCT2
• intestinal transporters: P-gp and BCRP
• liver transporters: OATP1B1, OATP1B3, P-gp, and BCRP
• kidney transporters: OAT1, OAT3, OCT2, MATE1, MATE2-K, and P-gp.

Resources
FDA Guidance for Industry: In Vitro Drug Interaction Studies — Cytochrome CYP Enzyme- and Transporter-Mediated Drug Interactions (2020).

For selected Human Drug Transporters, their properties, substrates and inhibitors refer to Sect. 3.5.

5.3.2   Do Transporters Affect Drug Absorption and Tissue Distribution?

Intestinal drug transporters P-gp and BCRP can reduce absorption for those compounds that are P-gp and/or BCRP substrates. Co-administration of inhibitors for these drug transporters can enhance drug absorption and increase the bioavailability. However, often the impact of transporters on oral bioavailability is limited due to saturation of efflux transporters at the intestinal membrane. Theoretically, low solubility drugs have a higher probability of showing a transporter based DDI, causing a change in oral bioavailability as lower solubility will prevent transporter saturation.

Different from passive diffusion, drug transporters can transport compounds against drug concentration gradients. Therefore, drug transporters can affect drug tissue distribution. Actually, P-gp is the major mechanism at the blood-brain barrier that prevents brain penetration of many compounds. Also, the efficacy of most statins is derived from their OATP-mediated uptake into the liver.

5.3.3 Can Drug Transporters Play an Important Role in Drug Clearance?

For BCS and BDDCS Class 3 and 4 compounds that have low membrane permeability, many are cleared as intact parent compounds in bile and urine with facilitation by drug transporters. Drug transporters can be the major driving force for clearance of these compounds.

References

Billington SS, Shoner S, Lee K et al (2019) Positron emission tomography imaging of [(11) C] Rosuvastatin hepatic concentrations and hepatobiliary transport in humans in the absence and presence of Cyclosporin a. Clin Pharmacol Ther 106:1056–1066

Cantrill C, Chaturvedi P, Rynn C, Petrig Schaffland J, Walter I, Wittwer MB (2020) Fundamental aspects of DMPK optimization of targeted protein degraders. Drug Discov Today 25(6):969–982

Fromm MF, Kim RB, Stein CM, Wilkinson GR, Roden DM (1999) Inhibition of P-glycoprotein-mediated drug transport: a unifying mechanism to explain the interaction between digoxin and quinidine. Circulation 99:552–557

Goetz GH, Philippe L, Shapiro MJ (2014) EPSA: a novel supercritical fluid chromatography technique enabling the design of permeable cyclic peptides. ACS Med Chem Lett 5(10):1167–1172

Hahn KK, Wolff JJ, Kolesar JM (2006) Pharmacogenetics and irinotecan therapy. Am J Health Syst Pharm 63:2211–2217

Hop CE (2006) Use of nano-electrospray for metabolite identification and quantitative absorption, distribution, metabolism and excretion studies. Curr Drug Metab 7(5):557–563. https://doi.org/10.2174/138920006777697909

Hop CE, Chen Y, Yu LJ (2005) Uniformity of ionization response of structurally diverse analytes using a chip-based nanoelectrospray ionization source. Rapid Commun Mass Spectrom 19(21):3139–3142. https://doi.org/10.1002/rcm.2182

Ma Y, Chen Y, Khojasteh SC, Dalvie K, Zhang D (2017) Glucuronides as anionic substrates of human CYP2C8. J Med Chem 60(21):8691–8705

Miners JO, McKinnon RA, Mackenzie PI (2002) Genetic polymorphisms of UDP-glucuronosyltransferases and their functional significance. Toxicology 181-182:453–456. https://doi.org/10.1016/s0300-483x(02)00449-3

Muller F, Weitz D, Mertsch K, Konig J, Fromm MF (2018) Importance of OCT2 and MATE1 for the cimetidine-metformin interaction: insights from investigations of polarized transport in single- and double-transfected MDCK cells with a focus on perpetrator disposition. Mol Pharm 15:3425–3433

Narang AS, Mahato RI (2010) Targeted delivery of small and macromolecular drugs, 1st edn. CRC Press. ISBN 9781138114517

Nguyen HQ, Kimoto E, Callegari E, Obach RS (2016) Mechanistic modeling to predict midazolam metabolite exposure from in vitro data. Drug Metab Dispos 44(5):781–791. https://doi.org/10.1124/dmd.115.068601. Epub 2016 Mar 8

O'Brien Z, Moghaddam MF (2015) A systematic analysis of physicochemical and ADME properties of all small molecule kinase inhibitors approved by US FDA from January 2001 to October 2015. Curr Med Chem 24(29):3159–3184. https://www.ncbi.nlm.nih.gov/pmc/articles/PMC5748879/

Schadt S, Chen L, Bischoff D (2011) Evaluation of relative LC/MS response of metabolites to parent drug in LC/Nanospray ionization mass spectrometry: potential implications in MIST assessment. J Mass Spectrom 46(12):1282–1287

Simonson SG, Raza A, Martin PD, Mitchell PD, Jarcho JA, Brown CD, Windass AS, Schneck DW (2004) Rosuvastatin pharmacokinetics in heart transplant recipients administered an antirejection regimen including cyclosporine. Clin Pharmacol Ther 76:167–177

Singh S, Bajpai M, Mishra P (2020) Self-emulsifying drug delivery system (SEDDS): an emerging dosage form to improve the bioavailability of poorly absorbed drugs. Crit Rev Ther Drug Carrier Syst 37:305–329

Takahashi RH, Khojasteh C, Wright M, Hop CECA, Ma S (2017) Mixed matrix method provides a reliable metabolite exposure comparison for assessment of metabolites in safety testing (MIST). Drug Metab Lett 11(1):21–28. https://doi.org/10.2174/1872312811666170710193229

Wang L, Raghavan N, He K, Luettgen JM, Humphreys WG, Knabb RM, Pinto DJ, Zhang D (2009) Sulfation of O-demethyl apixaban: enzyme identification and species comparison. Drug Metab Dispos 37(4):802–808

Zhang L, Wang S, Zhang M, Sun J (2013) Nanocarriers for oral drug delivery. J Drug Target 21:515–527

Zhang D, Hop CECA, Patilea-Vrana G et al (2019) Drug concentration asymmetry in tissues and plasma for small molecule-related therapeutic modalities. Drug Metab Dispos 47(10):1122–1135. https://doi.org/10.1124/dmd.119.086744. Epub 2019 Jul 2. PMID: 31266753; PMCID: PMC6756291

Zhang D, Wei C, Hop CECA et al (2021) Intestinal excretion, intestinal recirculation and renal tubulereabsorption are underappreciated mechanisms that drive the distribution and pharmacokinetic behavior of small molecule drugs. J Med Chem 64(11):7045–7059

Chapter 6
ADME Assays

Contents

Abstract The field of ADME sciences has seen the maturation and implementation of many predictive *in vitro* assays for small molecules over the past couple of decades. A survey in 1991 indicated that about 40% of all drugs in development failed because of poor ADME properties. It is very satisfying to see that the attrition in the clinic due to poor pharmacokinetic properties has decreased markedly. This can be ascribed to (1) high quality *in vitro* reagents and models, (2) bioanalytical advances and (3) integrated *in silico* models such as physiologically-based pharmacokinetic (PBPK) and pharmacokinetic/pharmacodynamics models.

These tools have allowed DMPK scientists to determine various key properties: (1) rates of metabolism (CL_{int}), (2) permeability, (3) drug transport, (4) drug metabolizing enzyme inhibition (mainly CYP and UGT enzymes), (5) tissue and plasma binding and (6) drug metabolizing enzyme regulation (induction). The combination of fast optimization of key DMPK properties based on a target profile together with efficient bioanalytical methods has allowed for robust screening of drug candidates.

© Springer Nature Switzerland AG 2022   175
S. C. Khojasteh et al., *Discovery DMPK Quick Guide*,
https://doi.org/10.1007/978-3-031-10691-0_6

For example, determining the metabolism rate *in vitro* using liver microsomes or hepatocytes has allowed for the calculation of *in vivo* clearance. The success of this and other assays has guided discovery teams to combine biological end points (i.e., potency and efficacy) with ADME properties.

Here we explore several of the major assays that are used during the drug discovery process. These assays can be performed using a variety of methods, and we will touch on the key concepts required to make the assays reliable and robust.

Keywords In vitro assays · Metabolism · Binding · Inhibition · Induction · Pharmacokinetics · Bioanalysis

Abbreviations

[S]	substrate concentration
AAG	α-acid glycoprotein
ABT	1-aminobenzotriazole
Acetyl CoA	Acetyl coenzyme A
AhR	Aryl hydrocarbon receptor
AI	Artificial Intelligence
AO	Aldehyde oxidase
APCI	Atmospheric pressure chemical ionization
API	Atmospheric pressure ionization
Caco-2	Human epithelial colorectal adenocarcinoma cells
CAR	Constitutively activated receptor
CES	Carboxylesterase
CHI	Chromatographic Hydrophobicity Index
CL_h	Predicted hepatic clearance
CL_{int}	Intrinsic clearance
CYP	Cytochrome P450
DDI	Drug-drug interaction
DME	Drug metabolizing enzymes
DMSO	Dimethyl sulfoxide
DNN	Deep neural network
ESI	Electrospray ionization
FMO	Flavin-containing monooxygenase
GLP	Good Laboratory Practice
GSH	Glutathione
HLM	Human liver microsomes
HPLC	High performance liquid chromatography
HSA	Human serum albumin
IAM	Immobilized artificial membranes
IS	Internal standard
Km	Michaelis-Menten constant
LC	Liquid chromatography

LM	Liver microsomes
MALDI	Matrix-assisted laser desorption/ionization
MDF	Mass defect filter
MIST	Metabolite in safety testing
MRM	Multiple reaction monitoring
MS	Mass spectrometry
NADH	Nicotinamide adenine dinucleotide (reduced form)
NADPH	Nicotinamide adenine dinucleotide phosphate (reduced form)
PAMPA	Parallel artificial membrane permeability assay
PAPS	3′-phosphoadenosine-5′-phosphosulfate
PBPK	Physiologically-based pharmacokinetic
PEG	Polyethylene glycol
PPB	Plasma protein binding
PXR	Pregnane X receptor
RF	Random forest
RM	Reactive metabolites
S9	Supernatant fraction derived by centrifugation of cell homogenate at 9000 g for 20 minutes
SFC	Supercritical fluid chromatography
SRM	Selected reaction monitoring
SVM	Support vector machine
$t_{1/2}$	Half-life
TDI	Time-dependent inhibition
TEER	Transepithelial electrical resistance
UDPGA	Uridine diphosphate glucuronic acid
UGT	Uridine 5′-diphospho-glucuronosyltransferase
UHPLC	Ultra high performance liquid chromatography

6.1   Overview of ADME Assays and Their Placement in the Discovery Cascade

A survey in 1991 indicated that about 40% of all drugs in development failed because of poor ADME properties (Kola and Landis 2004). It is very satisfying to see that the attrition in the clinic due to poor pharmacokinetic properties has decreased markedly. This can be ascribed to (1) high quality *in vitro* reagents and models, (2) bioanalytical advances and (3) integrated *in silico* models such as physiologically-based pharmacokinetic and pharmacokinetic/pharmacodynamics models.

ADME Challenges In modern day ADME assessment, several key assays are performed in parallel to determine a compound's potential liabilities. Other assays are gated based on the stage of the project. *In silico* models based on *in vitro* ADME data can be deployed prior to synthesis of compounds and more advanced *in silico* models, such as physiologically-based pharmacokinetic modeling, are often used later in drug discovery or in drug development to integrate a diverse set of data to make human predictions and minimize the use of resources.

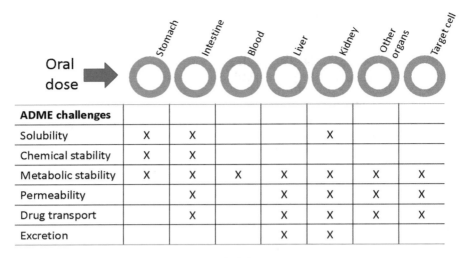

Fig. 6.1 ADME barriers for oral drugs to reach their target

Major ADME Barriers
Poor bioavailability and efficacy are usually observed for compounds with low solubility in the gastrointestinal tract, low permeability across cell membranes, and/or low chemical and metabolic stabilities (Fig. 6.1). As such, the three main properties that determine drug liabilities are:

1. Solubility
2. Permeability
3. Stability (both chemical and metabolic)

ADME Assays   *In vitro* assays to support small molecule discovery can be divided into eight general categories as shown in Fig. 6.2.

ADME assays can be conducted *in vitro*, *ex vivo* or *in vivo* (Table 6.1). *In vitro* assays are the most commonly used ADME model, followed by simple *in vivo* PK studies (Table 6.2). *Ex vivo* and more advanced *in vivo* studies are typically hypothesis-driven and are usually used to solve a specific issue.

Note that metabolism is frequently one of the major elimination pathways of drugs from the body (Table 6.3; Cerny 2016). Hepatic metabolic stability can, therefore, be a major ADME liability since a high rate of metabolism leads to a high intrinsic clearance (CL_{int}) and low exposure.

When major metabolic liabilities are not known, certain assumptions can be made appropriately evaluate the compound. *In silico* models have shown their power at predicting these properties and can lower the burden of laboratory-generated data.

Placement of Assays in the Discovery Cascade   The order in which ADME assays are conducted is dependent on a variety of factors including the therapeutic target,

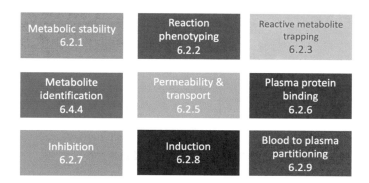

Fig. 6.2 Nine categories of *in vitro* assays used to support the discovery of small molecules

Table 6.1 Various types of ADME assessments and measurement in discovery stage

Type of study	Properties studied
Structural studies	logP, logD$_{7.4}$, pKa, PSA, MW, HBA, HBD
Chemical studies	Solubility Chemical stability
In vitro ADME	Permeability Stability (plasma, liver fractions, lysosomes) Metabolism (rates & sites) Inhibition (CYP & other enzymes) Induction (CYP & other enzymes) Plasma and tissue binding Transport (uptake/efflux) substrate/inhibition
In vivo PK	PK in rodent and non-rodent Bile-duct cannulated studies PK studies using inhibitors such as 1-aminobenzotriazole (ABT) Transgenic or humanized rodents

HBA hydrogen bond acceptor, *HBD* hydrogen bond donor, *logP* partition coefficient, *logD$_{7.4}$* partition coefficient at pH 7.4, *PSA* polar surface area

desired target coverage (concentration and time needed to elicit efficacy), route of administration, type of molecule (small molecule or other modality such as degraders or peptides), and relevant species.

Tiered ADME Assays
ADME assays can be separated into discovery phase and development phase assays. Discovery phase assays can be further classified as Tier 1, 2 or 3 (Table 6.4) at Genentech and other companies.

Tier 1 and 2 assays are established assays with known, reproducible and robust end points.

- Tier 1 assays are typically high throughput and can be requested by any member of the project team, though typically the medicinal chemists request them.

Table 6.2 Typical *in vitro*, *ex vivo* and *in vivo* models used to study metabolism, transport and excretion

Property	*In vitro*	*Ex vivo*	*In vivo*/PK
Metabolism	Liver microsome, hepatocyte, Cytosol	Liver or Intestinal perfusion	PK with chemical inhibitors such as ABT Bile-duct cannulated rat KO animal (P-gp, CYP, etc.)
Transport	Hepatocyte uptake		

ABT 1-aminobenzotriazole, *CYP* cytochrome P450, *KO* knock-out, *P-gp* P-glycoprotein

Table 6.3 Routes of elimination of marketed drugs from 2006 to 2015

Route of elimination	Percent of marketed drugs
Metabolism	
CYP	52%
UGT	12%
Hydrolase	11%
Carbonyl reductase	2.4%
Aldehyde oxidase	1.1%
Other	3.9%
No metabolism	18%

Cerny (2016)

Table 6.4 ADME assays that are typically conducted in Tiers 1, 2 and 3 during drug discovery

Tier	Assay
Tier 1	Liver microsomes (cross species), solubility, permeability
Tier 2	CYP inhibition (all major human CYPs) Time-dependent inhibition (all major human CYPs) Hepatocyte stability (cross species) Soft spot metabolite identification (cross species) Plasma protein binding (cross species) CYP induction (human only)
Tier 3 (hypothesis-driven)	Tissue binding (plasma in higher species, brain, tumor, etc.) Trapping assays using GSH, methoxylamine and cyanide Reaction phenotyping (CYP, UGT, AO, FMO) Metabolite identification

CYP cytochrome P450, *AO* aldehyde oxidase, *FMO* flavin-containing monooxygenase, *GSH* glutathione, *UGT* glucuronosyltransferase

- Tier 2 assays are requested by the ADME representative, and the generated data is combined with data from other assays. This allows for decision-making for the next set of compounds. Dependent on the known liability of a compound, specific assays can be placed in Tier 1 or 2. For example, if CYP inhibition is a potential liability, this assay will be placed in Tier 1 in order to quickly eliminate molecules that display potent inhibition. If CYP inhibition is not considered a liability, then this assay can be moved to Tier 2.

- Tier 3 assays are hypothesis-driven studies that are used to pinpoint specific liabilities that might not have been captured in the previous tiers. For example, UGT inhibition studies are usually not conducted on a regular basis, but studies can be designed to investigate this inhibition in a specific molecule if this liability is suspected.

6.2   *In Vitro* Assays

6.2.1   *Metabolic Stability*

This assay is used to determine the metabolic stability of a compound in an *in vitro* system that contains drug metabolizing enzymes (DME), most often CYP and UGT enzymes (see Tables 6.S.1 and 6.S.2 for a more comprehensive list). The most common matrices are liver microsomes (LM) or hepatocytes, but other alternatives such as cytosol, plasma, and cellular subcellular fractions derived from intestines or other tissues can be used depending upon the metabolic pathways of the chemical series. For low clearance compounds, a hepatocyte-relay method has been used to estimate the *in vitro* clearance value; in this assay, compounds are incubated with hepatocytes for a few hours and then the incubation mixture is centrifuged and fresh hepatocytes are administered to the supernatant and this cycle is repeated a few times.

Hepatocytes contain all hepatic enzymes and maintain the natural cellular architecture and functionalities of hepatic drug transporters. This matrix is, therefore, regarded as the most relevant *in vitro* system for most drugs for predicting *in vivo* intrinsic clearance and identifying the metabolites formed. The ease of use of hepatocytes has allowed for more-comprehensive metabolism assessments (including both Phase I and II DME) earlier in the discovery process. In many instances, DME activity depends on the presence of cofactors in the incubation (Table 6.S.1).

6.2.2   *The Metabolic Stability Assay*

Data Analysis
Samples are analyzed with LC-MS and peak areas for the test compound (parent) and the internal standard are measured and converted to the percent parent remaining and are calculated by normalizing the peak area ratio of parent to internal standard at t_0 (zero incubation time). Extra caution is needed to define t_0 for chemical reactive compounds. The observed rate constant (k_{obs}) for parent disappearance is calculated by determining the slope of the line of the graph of the natural log of percent parent remaining versus time of incubation.[66] Metabolic stability rate categories allow for establishing the liability of predicted hepatic clearance (CL_h) (Table 6.5).

Table 6.5 Categories for metabolic stability rates based on predicted hepatic clearance (CL_h)

Category	CL_h (mg/min/kg)				
	Human	Rat	Mouse	Dog	Monkey
Stable	<6.21	<16.6	<27	<9.27	<13.1
Moderate	6.21–14.5	16.6–38.6	27–63	9.27–21.6	13.1–30.5
Labile	>14.5	>38.6	>63	>21.6	>30.5

Categories are based on turnover rate: stable <30%, moderate 30–70%, labile >70%

Assay Considerations

Drug depletion is the most commonly used approach for determining *in vitro* metabolic clearance in drug discovery without any prior knowledge of its metabolic pathways. This approach, however, does not work for low clearance compounds. Additionally, some highly lipophilic compounds may exhibit an irregular time course as a result of inconsistent recovery caused by high non-specific binding to the matrix and/or the plastic surface of the incubation wells, resulting in erroneous clearance data. As a result, an in-well crashing approach using various organic solvents may be required to improve material recovery and data quality.

Data Interpretation

Even at optimal assay conditions, discrepancies are common in clearance data between the hepatocyte and LM assays because of a number of mechanistic differences, such as the physical cell membrane barrier, different metabolic pathways, cofactor concentration and depletion, latency of UGT enzymes in LM, different levels of free fraction, and drug efflux and transporter effects.

Supplemental Material

Tables 6.S.3, 6.S.4, 6.S.5, 6.S.6, and 6.S.7.

6.2.3 Reaction Phenotyping

The goal of metabolic reaction phenotyping is to identify the enzyme(s) involved in the formation of a specific metabolite. Until recently, the focus of this process was on CYP and UGT enzymes, but it now extends to other enzymes such as AO, FMO, and CES. Metabolic reaction phenotyping is most often performed with human enzymes rather than enzymes from preclinical species (Zientek and Youdim 2015).

The Reaction Phenotyping Assay As described in Fig. 6.3, metabolic reaction phenotyping is usually performed after major metabolites have already been identified. For CYP phenotyping, a common practice is to incubate the compound (1 μM) with both recombinant enzymes (rCYPs, 20–40 pM) or pooled human liver microsomes (HLM, 0.5 mg/mL) in the absence or presence of isoform-specific chemical CYP inhibitors at their effective concentrations (Table 6.5). Phenotyping can also be

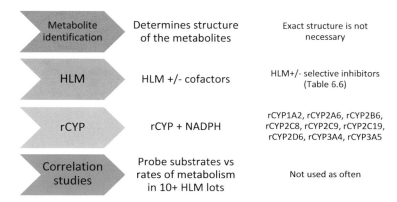

Fig. 6.3 Studies performed for metabolic reaction phenotyping

performed for other drug metabolizing enzymes, such as UGTs, AO, FMO and CES, but is less common. Hepatocytes is also used in reaction phenotyping.

Data Analysis
The relative rate of depletion of the test compound and formation of its metabolites by individual recombinant CYP (rCYP) enzymes can be determined by measuring the corresponding peak area ratios of the test compound (parent) and its metabolite relative to the peak area of the internal standard using LC-MS. Subsequently, both depletion and formation rate for each CYP isoform are normalized according to its relative abundance in human liver.

Similarly, inhibitory effects of isoform specific inhibitors44 on drug depletion and metabolite formation in HLM can be determined by measuring the corresponding peak area ratios of the test compound (parent) and its metabolite relative to that of the control (no inhibitor).

Assay Considerations
HLM is widely used for CYP-related reaction phenotyping. For drug candidates with both CYP and non-CYP mediated metabolism, however, human hepatocytes in combination with enzyme specific chemical inhibitors can be the preferred *in vitro* system for reaction phenotyping in order to estimate the relative contribution of individual metabolic pathways. Cytosolic fractions can be considered when phenotyping AO, FMO, and CES enzymes. Additionally, it is good practice to confirm the results using recombinant enzymes.

Data Interpretation
The highest depletion rate by a specific rCYP indicates that this enzyme has the largest contribution to the overall metabolism of the test compound. This should be in agreement with the rate of metabolite formation by the same rCYP. Likewise, drug depletion and metabolite formation in HLM should be slowed down the most by the corresponding inhibitor. However, when hepatocytes are used for reaction phenotyping, precaution must be taken in data interpretation given the fact that

Table 6.6 Chemical inhibitors and inactivators used in reaction phenotyping assays

CYP	Inhibitor/inactivator (μM)
1A2	Furafylline (10): **Ia**
2B6	2-Phenyl-2-(1-piperidinyl)propane (20): **I**
2C8	Montelukast (2): **I**
2C9	Sulfaphenazole (10): **I**
2C19	(+)-*N*-3-Benzylnirvanol (2): **I**
2D6	Quinidine (1): **I**
3A	Ketoconazole (1): **I**; Troleandomycin (20): **Ia**
Broad	1-Aminobenzotriazole (ABT; 1000): **Ia**

I inhibitor, *Ia* inactivator. Pre-incubation is required for inactivators

multiple metabolic pathways can occur and a potential compensatory mechanism may exist between different metabolic pathways in the presence of inhibitors (Table 6.6).

6.2.4 Reactive Metabolite Trapping Studies

Trapping assays are used to assess the formation of reactive metabolites (RM) that can be formed as a result of bioactivation (i.e., the process of metabolism). RM has the potential to react and form adducts with various macromolecules (proteins, DNA, etc.) and may, therefore, result in toxicity (Schadt et al. 2015). Trapping assays use various nucleophiles to 'trap' RM, which then stabilizes the RM and allows for detection of the conjugates. These assays are predominantly conducted in liver microsome incubations fortified with NADPH and glutathione (GSH).

6.2.4.1 Chemical Trapping Agents

GSH Conjugates
GSH conjugates are suited for the detection of soft electrophiles such as Michael acceptors and epoxides. To screen for GSH conjugates use the following:

- 129 Da (glutamic acid) neutral loss scan in the positive ion mode on MS/MS
- m/z 272 precursor ion scan in the negative ion mode on MS/MS (Yan and Caldwell 2004)

The detection of GSH conjugates is more selective when using a mixture of regular and stable labeled GSH (Yan and Caldwell 2004).

GSH Analogs
GSH detection by LC-MS/MS is not quantitative, and other trapping analogs such as [³H]GSH and dansyl-GSH (Gan et al. 2005) can be used for this purpose.

In addition, quaternary ammonium GSH analogs produce more-sensitive GSH adducts (Soglia et al. 2006) and peptides (Wei et al. 2013) have been used as well. Note that analogs of GSH are not catalyzed by glutathione *S*-transferase (GST).

Cyanide Conjugates
Cyanide conjugates are suitable for the detection of iminium ions. To screen for cyanide conjugates use:

- 27 Da neutral loss scan in the positive ion mode on a triple quadrupole mass spectrometer (Argoti et al., 2005). A mixture of CN^- and stable labeled $^{13}C^{15}N^-$ enhances the selectivity for detection of cyanide conjugates.

Methoxylamine and Semicarbazide Conjugates
These conjugates are suitable for trapping aldehydes. No straightforward fragmentation pattern exists for MS/MS methods in any scan mode for automated data acquisition.

Covalent Modification of Proteins   The covalent binding of drugs to endogenous biomolecules, such as proteins, has been determined for many years, and higher-throughput methods have been established (Day et al. 2005). Some companies have integrated covalent binding assays into the drug discovery stage and, although no fixed cut-off values are broadly applicable, a value of >50 pmol/mg protein is proposed as the threshold beyond which the drug candidate should not be pursued further (Evans et al. 2004). However, evaluation requires the availability of radiolabeled analogs, which may be hard and time-consuming to synthesize. When multiple radiolabeled compounds are available, structure–activity relationships can be generated, potentially leading to the development of drugs that reduce or eliminate the extent of covalent binding. Note, however, that no apparent quantitative link exists between covalent binding and toxicity (Obach et al. 2008).

6.2.5   Metabolite Identification

The objectives of metabolite identification in the discovery stage are to:

1. Identify metabolic soft spots (types of metabolites: Phase I and II)
2. Determine the enzymes that generate the metabolite
3. Compare *in vitro* metabolism across species
4. Screen for reactive metabolite
5. Identify circulating metabolites (that can be relatively inert, active or cause toxicity)

Note: Metabolite-in-safety testing (MIST) considerations are out of scope during the discovery stage. The first considerations on metabolites comes from the metabolites formed in hepatocytes. This is opportunity to examine if primary and secondary metabolites could potentially be absent in species used as toxicology models. The second opportunity is when examining preclinical circulating metabolites. If circulating metabolites are observed in preclinical species, chances are high that MIST will be considered due to the relatively higher dose required in preclinical tox studies. The existence of active metabolites (on or off target) that contribute to the pharmacology and/or toxicity can be a reason to monitor the metabolites.

Methods of Metabolite Identification   Most metabolites are from expected metabolic pathways such as oxidation, glucuronidation, or demethylation (M + 16, M + 176, M-14) by common DMEs. These metabolites can be easily identified with the mass spectrometry vendor metabolite processing software. Identification of uncommon metabolites (with unpredicted molecular weights) remains challenging. Identification of all metabolites can be accomplished with the following techniques.

Mass Defect Filter (MDF)
The mass defects of common metabolic reactions are generally less than 50 mDa of the parent drug decimal mass. MDF removes non-drug-related ions whose mass defects lie outside of this window using high resolution MS data.

Background Subtraction
This method uses accurate mass data coupled with retention-time-shift tolerance to determine if an ion detected in the analyte file is present in the control file (e.g., t_0 incubation).

Isotope-Pattern-Filtering
This technique facilitates the detection of metabolites that possess highly diagnostic isotopic patterns (*e.g.*, chlorine- and bromine-containing compounds) that fall within 5 ppm tolerance.

Chemical Derivatization
Derivatization is a technique used to modify the potential site of modification with a specific functional group (Liu and Hop 2005). Ideally, derivatization should be a one-step process without purification that can be performed at the bench with limited synthetic chemistry skills.

H/D Exchange
This is a reaction in which exchangeable hydrogen atoms in a compound (or a metabolite) are replaced with deuterium. This is done by performing the reaction/incubation in D_2O instead of H_2O. D_2O does not need to be 100% pure but the percent incorporation is calculated based on %D_2O. Changes in the molecular weight of molecular ions and fragment ions that contain exchanged hydrogen atoms are detected by MS. Note that if the samples are run in a mobile phase with H_2O, exchangeable deuterium atoms will most likely be replaced back to hydrogen. To avoid this, a direct infusion can be carried out or D_2O can be used in the mobile phase.

Chromatographic Hydrophobicity Index (CHI)   LC retention could allow better estimation of site of metabolism (Fitch et al. 2018).

Supplemental Material
Table 6.S.8

6.2.6   Permeability and Transport

Permeability is one of the key factors determined in the compound evaluation. This allows for a better understanding of whether a compound can be absorbed and reach intracellular targets as well as all other influences permeability has on other ADME properties. Hand in hand with permeability assessment is an understanding of the role of drug transport in assisting molecules in crossing cellular membranes. Several assays are deployed for this purpose.

In Vitro Permeability Assays
Parallel Artificial Membrane Permeability Assay (PAMPA). This assay is used to determine passive phospholipid permeation. Transwell format plates are used. This assay is compatible with a large range of pH on either side of the membrane, which may otherwise not be achieved using cells.
Immobilized Artificial Membranes (IAM). This is a chromatography-based analysis that examines the molecular interactions between phospholipids bound to silica on a column (Luco et al. 2003). This is amenable to high throughput analysis and could be a reasonable descriptor for permeability.
Supercritical Fluid Chromatography (EPSA). This is another chromatography-based assay using supercritical fluid chromatography and could be a good descriptor of polar surface area (Goetz et al. 2014). Currently, this method is applied to larger molecules such as macrocyclic peptides.

Human Epithelial Colorectal Adenocarcinoma Cells (Caco-2) This was the first cell line used for the assessment of intestinal absorption (Sambuy et al. 2005), and the application of this model can be expanded to capture cellular permeability. The confluent cells are differentiated and represent mature enterocytes that are polarized with transporters to reflect natural biology. Notably, the metabolic competency of these cells for oxidation by CYP is limited. In addition, paracellular (between cells) versus transcellular (through cell) pathways must be considered. Due to the polar surface area and molecular size, the major pathway is usually transcellular for most small molecules. However, at times due to cytotoxicity or generation of tight junction gaps, the paracellular pathway becomes important.

Lucifer yellow (detected by fluorescence) or trans-epithelial electrical resistance (TEER) can be used to examine the integrity and permeability of the cell monolayer.

Madin Darby Canine Kidney (MDCK) This is another popular cell-based permeability tool. One advantage of MDCK over Caco2 is the decreased amount of time required to wait after seeding to generate an intact monolayer of cells to perform the permeability assay. Notably, drug transport differences exist between the two cell lines, such as p-gp expression in dog versus human. However, certain transporters can be knocked out to remove them from the cells.

Transwell Assays
These assays involve two chambers that are separated by a microporous membrane, with cells growing in the upper chamber. The cells need to be confluent in order to assure that compounds permeating from one chamber to another are required to pass through the cells.

In Vitro **Drug Transporter Assays**   In these assays, drug transporters are overexpressed in cell lines and the interaction of test compounds with the transporters is measured. Whether a test compound is an inhibitor or substrate of a specific transporter can affect the distribution and overall PK of the drug.

Drug transporter substrates and inhibitors *in vitro see* Table 3.15.

ATPase Assay – A membrane assay that indirectly measures activity of the transporter of interest. The transport of substrates for ABC transporters requires ATP hydrolysis. ATP hydrolysis results in the release of inorganic phosphate, which can be measured using simple colorimetric analysis.

Membrane Vesicle Assay – Inverted plasma membrane vesicles have been used to study transport. Cell lines used to prepare membrane vesicles include drug selected cells, transfected cells and baculovirus infected insect cells. As the membranes are inverted, influx rather than efflux is used to measure transporter activity. Using this system, detailed kinetic experiments can be performed. Activity of ABC transporters have been studied using this type of assay.

Cell lines – Polarized cell line assays, where the flux of compound from apical to basolateral and basolateral to apical is measured, are commonly used to study transport and permeability. Cell lines used in this type of assay include Caco-2 (human epithelial colorectal adenocarcinoma cells) and MDCK (Madin-Darby canine kidney cells) cells. The expression of transporters in Caco-2 cells is comparable to that observed in the small intestine. In contrast, endogenous expression of transporters in MDCK cells is low. In addition, as MDCK cells are derived from dog, transporters expressed will be of dog origin.

Transfected Cell Lines – Transfected cell lines contain recombinant transporters that are either stably or transiently expressed. Transfections can be single or double and can include efflux and/or uptake transporters. Cell lines used for transfection include MDCK, LLC-PK1, HEK 293 or CHO cells. An example of a commonly used transfected cell line is MDR1 transfected MDCKII cells for the study of P-gp.

Primary Cells – Primary cells in some cases can be isolated from intact tissue and will contain the full complement of transporters present in the tissue of interest. Primary cells will adapt to culture condition quickly and transporter expression can change. An example of a primary cell assay is the brain microvessel endothelial cell assay. Properties of primary cells in culture must be understood prior to deploying the assay.

Hepatocyte in Sandwich Culture – A hepatocyte sandwich culture assay involves culturing hepatocytes between two layers of gelled collagen. Hepatocytes in this configuration have the ability to form bile canaliculi and have a full complement of hepatic transporters on sinusoidal and canalicular membranes. Thus, this type of assay has been used to investigate biliary clearance of drugs.

In Vivo **Assessment of Drug Transport** Leveraging humanized animal models to understand human drug disposition is captured in a publication by Choo and Salphati (2018). Knockout and transgenic knockin models and naturally occurring transporter deficient animal models are useful tools to understand the *in vivo* contribution of transporters. An example of the use of knockout animal studies to investigate the role of transporters in *in vivo* disposition is the use of *Mdr 1a*$^{-/-}$ mice to demonstrate the role of P-gp in limiting brain exposure. Despite the advantages of using *in vivo* systems to investigate transporters, there are limitations to these *in vivo* models. Alterations in the expression of transporters and enzymes can occur in knockout and knockin animals. In addition, the level of expression of transporters can sometimes differ between animals and humans. These factors need to be considered when interpreting the results from studies using knockout and knockin animals.

6.2.7 Plasma Protein Binding

Determination of the unbound fraction in plasma or various tissues allows for the prediction of DDI potential, *in vivo* clearance, efficacy, and toxicity risks because it is the unbound drug that interacts with macromolecular targets.

Plasma Protein Binding Assays Three commonly used methods for PPB determination are equilibrium dialysis (ED) (Waters et al. 2008), ultrafiltration (UF) (Wang and Williams 2013), and ultracentrifugation (UC). The advantages and disadvantages of each method are summarized in Table 6.7. ED is generally regarded as the preferred method since it is truly based on drug equilibrium between plasma proteins and buffer across a semipermeable membrane. Also, the ED method is easy to adapt for both automation and higher throughput.

Leakage of the Membrane Can Sometimes Occur in the ED and UF Methods and, Therefore, Use of One or More Positive Controls is Suggested
The pH of the plasma needs to be buffered since plasma becomes more basic over time and this can impact the f_u of basic drugs.

The unbound drug fraction needs to be soluble in the buffer compartment.

Solvent concentrations should be minimized since solvents can interfere with binding to plasma proteins and increase the free fraction.

Note that the f_u can be influenced by free fatty acids.

Table 6.7 Comparison of three methods for determining plasma protein binding

	Equilibrium dialysis (ED)	Ultrafiltration (UF)	Ultracentrifugation (UC)
Mechanism of separation	Semipermeable membranes Time to equilibrium = 4–24 h (for highly bound compounds)	Semipermeable membranes Centrifugation at 2000xg Analyze 10–50 filterates	Layer formation of plasma components Centrifugation at 625,000xg
Advantages	Higher throughput	Fast Higher throughput	Medium throughput
Disadvantages	Volume shift Leakage of the membrane Non-specific binding Donnan effect based on charge	Leakage of the membrane Non-specific binding Donnan effect	Increasing pH during centrifugation Lacks complete layer formation Samples must be taken shortly after stopping centrifugation Requirement of high speed centrifuge
Practical notes	Teflon plates minimize non-specific binding	Easy and fast	Top layer lipid interference

Data Analysis

When ED is used for PPB, the fraction unbound (f_u) in matrix is calculated from taking the ratio of response on the receiver side to response on the donor side. The ratios are normalized to the internal standard peak areas (Chen et al. 2018). The percent protein binding is the inverse of f_u.

$$ f_\mathrm{u} = \frac{\left[\dfrac{analyte\,peak\,area,\,buffer}{IS\,peak\,area,\,buffer} \right]}{\left[\dfrac{analyte\,peak\,area,\,plasma}{IS\,peak\,area,\,plasma} \right]} $$

Assay Considerations

Although the PPB assay is straightforward, f_u values can be variable due to a number of reasons including the physicochemical properties of the test compound and assay conditions such as salt concentration, buffering strength, and pH range in dialysis buffer. Additionally, the length of incubation (6–24 hr) is critical to ensure that true equilibrium is achieved in the ED assay; this is especially important for compounds with a high logD value and slow diffusion rate across the semipermeable membrane. For highly bound compounds (>99% bound), diluted plasma (10%) can be used to determine $f_\mathrm{u,d}$, which can then be extrapolated to the value in undiluted plasma according to the equation below:

$$f_u = \frac{1/D}{\left[\left(\dfrac{1}{fu,d}\right)-1\right]+1/D}$$

It is highly recommended that low f_u values (< 0.01) are confirmed using an orthogonal approach (Chen et al. 2018) because of concerns regarding incomplete equilibrium and the potential impact of non-specific binding. Similarly, diluted plasma can be also used for labile compounds to slow down drug depletion due to metabolism in plasma and facilitate equilibrium (Leung et al. 2020).

Data Interpretation
In human plasma, drugs can bind to both serum albumin (HSA ~670 µM) and α-acid glycoprotein (AAG ~20 µM). For the majority drugs, f_u values are usually comparable when measured at different concentrations. However, a higher f_u value can be observed if a drug predominantly binds to AAG and binding saturation occurs at high drug concentrations. Binding saturation may also occur when diluted plasma ($< 5\%$) is used and the drug concentration is relatively high. In general, the impact of drug recovery on f_u is minimal as long as true equilibrium is achieved in the assay.

6.2.8   Drug Metabolizing Enzyme Inhibition

Inhibition assays assess the potential for drug-drug interactions (DDIs) that are caused by the inhibition of DMEs, mainly CYP enzymes followed by UGT1A1, or drug transporters. Enzyme inhibition can be either reversible or irreversible/time-dependent.

The Reversible Enzyme Inhibition Assay The test compound is incubated at various concentrations with human liver microsomes (HLM) fortified with NADPH and a CYP isoform-specific probe substrate (Khojasteh et al. 2011). The specific concentrations of HLM and probe substrates as well as the length of incubation are optimized to ensure that incubations are within the linear range of metabolite formation for each probe substrate (Table 6.8). Reactions are terminated by protein precipitation, and samples are prepared for LC-MS analysis to monitor CYP activity by determining the extent of metabolite formation of the probe substrates. The metabolite formation at various concentrations of test compound is compared to a vehicle control containing no test compound. Any decrease in the amount of metabolite formed when a test compound is present is indicative of CYP inhibition. The concentration of test compound and amount of metabolite formed are used to calculate an IC_{50} value (concentration at which the test compound inhibits 50% of the enzyme activity).

Table 6.8 Typical selective CYP substrates and metabolites monitored

CYP	Probe substrate	[S] (μM)	Metabolite monitored	Time (min)	HLM (mg/ml)
1A2	Phenacetin	50	Acetaminophen	30	0.03
2B6	Buproprion	80	Hydroxybupropion	20	0.05
2C8	Paclitaxel	4	6α-hydroxypaclitaxel	8	0.05
2C9	(S)-warfarin	2	7-hydroxywarfarin	30	0.2
2C19	(S)-mephenytoin	60	4′-hydroxymephenytoin	40	0.2
2D6	Dextromethorphan	5	Dextrorphan	10	0.03
3A	Testosterone	50	6β-hydroxytestosterone	10	0.07
3A	Midazolam	2	1′-hydroxymidazolam	10	0.03

Data Analysis

To determine IC_{50} values, the ratio of peak area to internal standard of each CYP-specific metabolite is quantified for each concentration of test compound. The percent remaining activity is plotted against the concentration of inhibitor, and IC_{50} values can be calculated by non-linear regression using the following equation:

$$Y = 100 / \left(1 + 10 \wedge X - \log\left(IC_{50}\right)\right)$$

Assay Considerations

It is a common practice to pool assay samples prior to LC-MS/MS analysis to increase the assay throughput, but it is important to achieve sufficient chromatographic separations in order to avoid potential interference of the test compound with the response of CYP-specific metabolites. This interference produces a false reading since it may appear that less metabolite has been formed as a result of ion suppression of the CYP-specific metabolite by the test compound when it co-elutes with the CYP probe metabolite at a relatively high concentration. Keeping in mind the sensitivity of analytical detection, low microsomal protein concentrations are preferred to minimize the effort of drug binding to the matrix, and short incubation times are recommended to avoid potential substrate depletion. For low solubility compounds, a proper organic solvent is required to achieve sufficient coverage for C_{max} without potential inhibitory effects on CYP activity.

Data Interpretation

It is not uncommon to observe an atypical dose response curve for a low solubility compound due to precipitation in the serial dilution. Also, inhibition potency or IC_{50} values of a given compound can differ when two different substrates are used for the same CYP isoform, as can happen with CYP3A4 or CYP2C9. Additionally, an increase of CYP activity by the test compound can occasionally be observed. This is known as an allosteric effect of the compound on the enzyme that results from a conformational change involving protein–drug binding dynamics, which can eventually lead to an increase in enzyme activity. Test compounds can be classified into three general categories according to IC_{50} value of CYP inhibition: potent (< 1 μM), moderate (1–10 μM), and weak (>10 μM). Finally, the risk of drug-drug interaction in the clinic has to be viewed in light of the human drug concentration of the test compound, including C_{max}. Indeed, a moderately potent CYP inhibitor can still result in significant DDI if the systemic concentrations of the test compound are very high. While these CYP inhibition studies can provide a general idea of DDI potential, more robust data interpretation and better DDI prediction should be made using static or PBPK models.

Time-Dependent CYP Inhibition Irreversible CYP inhibition by test compounds can be determined in the presence of hepatic drug metabolizing enzymes in liver microsomes using concentration ranges up to the highest concentration allowed by solubility (Mukadam et al. 2012). The test compound is incubated at a wide range of concentrations (typically: 0 (vehicle control), 0.1, 1, 5, and 10 µM) during a pre-incubation in LM plus NADPH. In the second step, the incubation mixture is diluted ten-fold (or more) and incubated with CYP-probes (typically at K_m). The reaction is quenched by solvent containing a stable-labeled internal standard and then analyzed by LC-MS for metabolite formation.

Data Analysis
Peak area ratios are calculated by dividing the peak area of each probe metabolite by the respective stable-labelled IS peak area. Percent activity is calculated by normalizing peak area ratios of samples containing test compound to vehicle controls. A shift in the IC50 in the presence or absence of NADPH in the pre-incubation are captured as follow.

$$AUC\,shift\,(\%) = 100 \times \left(1 - \frac{AUC + NADPH}{AUC - NADPH} \right)$$

Time-Dependent Inhibition (K_I and k_{inact} Determination) This assay is conducted as further examination to determine the maximal rates of enzyme inactivation (k_{inact}) and the inhibitor concentration leading to half maximal inactivation (K_I) of a test compound in the presence of hepatic drug metabolizing enzymes. While time-dependent CYP inhibition is assessed in drug discovery, definitive determination of K_I and k_{inact} is usually performed in the development stage. k_{obs} is the negative slope of the initial phase of inactivation and can be calculated by:

$$k_{obs} = \frac{[I] \times k_{inact}}{[I] + K_I}$$

where [I] is the test compound concentration. The k_{obs} is determined by a linear fit of the natural logarithm of percent control activity versus time for each test compound concentration.

Cut-off values to indicate weak inhibition are used to avoid reporting unnecessary alarming? values. A greater than 25% loss of control activity at the earliest pre-incubation time is considered to be extensive reversible inhibition. All concentrations meeting this criterion are excluded from k_{obs} calculations so that only time-dependent inhibition is considered. In addition, a less than 20% loss of control activity over the longest pre-incubation time is classified as non-quantifiable (kinetic parameters cannot be accurately defined because <20% loss is within the range of assay and quantification variability).

pHep Assay In this assay, suspended human hepatocytes are incubated with human plasma and the test compound. CYP3A inhibition is measured along with TDI and reversible inactivation (Mao et al. 2012).

Assay Considerations
Similar to the reversible CYP inhibition assay, one must be mindful about the potential impact of hepatocyte concentrations, solvents and insufficient chromatographic separations. For compounds with low solubility or high incubation binding, a non-diluted method can be used instead. For compounds with high reversible inhibition potency, the pre-incubation time and the fold of dilution deserve special consideration in order to avoid potential false negatives.

Data Interpretation
The sensitivity of a CYP TDI assay can be enzyme substrate dependent (midazolam vs testosterone for CYP3A4). It is important to note that CYP TDI can be caused by either irreversible binding of a drug to the enzyme or inhibition by a more potent metabolite, and differentiation between the two mechanisms can be of significance in clinical DDI prediction. Additionally, it has recently been reported that covalent inhibitors can exhibit NADPH independent time-dependent CYP inhibition due to chemical reactivity to the enzyme (Kosaka et al. 2020), which may lead to false negatives in a regular TDI assay.

6.2.9   Drug Metabolizing Enzyme Induction

Induction studies are used to investigate the potential induction of a test compound against DME (mainly CYP enzymes) in human cryopreserved hepatocytes and enterocytes. The mechanisms of induction are complex, but these three receptors (listed in order of importance) play a major role[81]: pregnane X receptor (PXR), constitutively activated receptor (CAR), and aryl hydrocarbon receptor (AhR). These regulatory elements control many Phase I and II DME in addition to drug transporters (Table 6.9). Typically, primary hepatocytes are used to capture all the relevant induction risks during the discovery stage.

The Induction Assay Cells are plated on collagen-coated plates and allowed to equilibrate for several days before treatment. The positive control, vehicle control or test compounds are dosed on day 2–3 for 48–72 hours, with the medium changed every 24 hours. Enzyme activity is determined after 72 hours incubations using the probe substrates phenacetin for CYP1A2, bupropion for CYP2B6, and testosterone for CYP3A4 (Table 6.9). Samples are analyzed by LC-MS/MS to quantify formation of the metabolites. In addition, mRNA levels of the DMEs are deteremined from

Table 6.9 List of drug metabolizing enzymes and drug transporters that are induced by nuclear receptors (Hewitt et al. 2008)

Nuclear receptor	Phase I	Phase II	Drug transporter
Pregnane X receptor (PXR)	CYP2B, CYP2C, **CYP3A4**, CYP7A	UGT1A1, GST-A2	MDR1, MRP2, OATP2, OCT1
Constitutively activated receptor (CAR)	**CYP2B6**, CYP3A, CYP2A	UGT1A1, SULT1A1	MRP3, MRP2, OATP2
Aryl hydrocarbon receptor (**AhR**)	CYP1A1, CYP1A2, CYP1B1, ALDH	UGT1A1, SULT1A1, GST-A2	MDR1

these samples and so is cell viability to ensure that the effects are not caused by cell toxicity. Usually, the cells are lysed after 48 h incubations to quantitate mRNA levels (Halladay et al. 2012; Kenny et al. 2018).

Assay Considerations
It is widely recognized that the results of the CYP induction assay are quite variable from run to run even when the assay is performed by the same scientist; dramatic variability is often observed between different donors. The variability in data is partly due to the dynamic nature of the assay readouts (mRNA and enzyme activity). It is critical to keep assay conditions consistent including cell density, seeding and inducing time, and post-assay incubation with CYP substrates. Usually, a more sensitive donor can be used for initial screening of CYP induction. If the induction data is intended for DDI prediction, the initial screen is followed by a more stringent assay using multiple donors to better manage the impact of donor differences. Additionally, measuring the actual concentration of the inducer at the end of incubation is suggested in order to contextualize the intrinsic induction potency of the drug. For cytotoxic compounds, a short incubation time (4–12 h) and lower drug concentrations should be considered.

Data Interpretation
EC_{50} and E_{max} are two key parameters required for DDI prediction; however, reliable results are not always feasible for these parameters. A bell-shaped curve can sometimes be observed for compounds with low solubility and/or high cytotoxicity of the test compound. Alternatively, the slope of the dose response curve may be used for assessing DDI potential. Additionally, an increase in CYP mRNA levels can be observed without an actual change in CYP activity if a test compound is both an inducer and a time dependent inhibitor of the same isoform. Similar results can also be obtained for a very potent reversible inhibitor as a result of residual contamination after changing of the medium. Finally, an increase in mRNA levels without a change in CYP activity can occur if a test compound blocks translation of mRNA to its corresponding CYP enzyme, a process which has been documented but is very rare. Regardless, DDI caused by CYP induction is much less common in the clinic than that caused by CYP inhibition.

6.2.10   Blood to Plasma Partitioning

Ivy Kekessi and Emile Plise
Blood to plasma partitioning (BPP) is a distribution assay for the quantification of
drug concentrations in pharmacokinetic (PK), safety, and/or efficacy studies. This
ADME parameter, often measured from the derived plasma, is critical for the evaluation of the drug's development potential and its pharmacokinetic/pharmacodynamic
properties (see Chap. 4). Careful consideration needs to be taken in assessing drug
concentrations from plasma versus the whole blood, as some compounds have a
greater affinity for red blood cells (RBC) compared to plasma (called sequestered to
the RBC), hence resulting in a possible misrepresentation of drug clearance (Dash
et al. 2021). For example, in the case romifidine (anaesthetic drug used in horses),
it was found to sequester to RBC compared to plasma (Romagnoli et al. 2017).
These findings indicate continuous and consistent release of romifidine from RBC
to plasma over the sedation period.

Data Analysis
Blood to plasma partition ratio (R) is determined at steady-state equilibrium by
determining the compound concentration in blood and the concentration of the
compound in the plasma obtained after the blood sample was centrifuged:

$$R = C_b / C_0$$

Where:
C_b = compound concentration in blood.
C_p = compound concentration in plasma collected by centrifuging the
blood sample.
The depletion method for determining the red blood cell partitioning ratio
(KRBC/PL) uses a plasma reference containing the same concentration of test compound as the whole blood sample. After centrifugation of the whole blood, plasma
is collected and analyzed along with the plasma reference samples. KRBC/PL is
calculated using the equation:

$$KRBC / PL = 1 / H \times (PLref / PLwb - 1) + 1$$

Where:
PLref = ratio of analyte to internal standard in the plasma reference.
PLwb = ratio of analyte to internal standard in plasma obtained from the whole
blood sample.
H = hematocrit.

Assay Considerations
Avoiding hemolysis of RBCs is essential for a successful partitioning experiment.
Fresh blood harvested immediately before the experiment is ideal. Alternatively,
properly refrigerated blood may be used up to 24 hours after collection. DMSO or

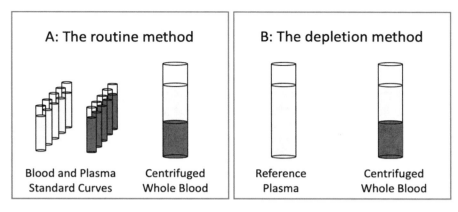

Fig. 6.4 Two schemes that captures the routine and the depletion methods. (**a**) for the routine method, the compound concentration is determined in the plasma and whole blood whole blood at the end of the incubation using the appropriate standard curve matrix, and (**b**) for the depletion method, the compound to the internal standard ratio is determined in the plasma reference and plasma obtained from the whole blood at the end of the incubation

other solvents concentrations should be kept to a minimum ($\leq 0.1\%$), while shaking and incubation time for the experiment should be optimized to ensure proper mixing and avoiding hemolysis. BPP may be saturable for some compounds, therefore best practice is to select a concentration or range of concentrations that cover the compound levels observed in PK studies. A typical BPP experiment should include a compound stability test and proper stability controls (*e.g.,* procaine) to ensure the enzymes in the blood are active and the test compounds are stable over the duration of the experiment. Drugs such as methazolamide, chloroquine, or chlorthalidone can be used as positive controls for partitioning into RBCs, and a negative control such as metoprolol that partitions equally between RBCs and plasma is recommended.

Analysis of the samples whether LC-MS/MS for non-labeled compounds (The routine method; Figure 6.4a) or liquid scintillation counting (LSC) for radiolabeled molecules have specific considerations (*e.g.* ^{14}C-labeled vismodegib; Wong et al. 2009). The anticoagulant heparin may cause suppression of LC-MS/MS signal. Therefore, alternatives such as EDTAK2 or K3 may be preferred. In the standard BPP assay, RBCs must be lysed completely to avoid coagulation and consistently extract the test compounds from the matrix. For radiolabeled compounds, an LSC may be prone to quenching due to the red color of blood, hence an LSC-compatible tissue solubilizer is recommended to lyse RBCs followed by a decolorizing step using bleach or hydrogen peroxide.

An additional method is the depletion method which is compatible with a high throughput discovery setting using LC-MS/MS (Fig. 6.4b; Yu et al., 2005).

Data Interpretation

An *in vitro* blood to plasma ratio of 0.8–1.2 suggests the affinity between the RBCs and plasma compartments is approximately equal; therefore, compound concentrations in plasma samples collected *in vivo* may be used to calculate pharmacokinetic (PK) parameters such as plasma clearance (CL_p). However, if the blood to plasma ratio is significantly greater than 1 *in vitro*, this may indicate the compound preferentially partitions into the erythrocytes and can lead to an overprediction of *in vivo* *CLp*. Where the ratio is greater than 1, either whole blood should be analyzed to obtain accurate PK parameters. Additionally, plasma may be analyzed in PK experiments if corrected by the blood plasma ratio. Blood to plasma ratios less than (< 0.7) indicate the compound mostly resides in the plasma compartment or equilibration in the in vitro partition assay was not achieved.

6.3   *In Vivo* Pharmacokinetics

For preclinical PK studies, for the sole purpose of PK evaluation, typically low doses are used in order to stay within the range where pharmacokinetics is linear and to reduce the amount of material that is consumed. Typical doses for preclinical pharmacokinetic studies are: 0.5 to 1 mg/kg for the intravenous route or 2 to 5 mg/kg for the oral route. PK studies whose purpose is to provide support for preclinical efficacy or toxicity studies may involve higher doses. These studies are performed to identify concentrations associated with an efficacious or toxic effect and may not be relevant to the lower doses that are ultimately administered to patients. Higher dose ranges in these studies can lead to saturation of metabolism resulting in a higher bioavailability when compared to lower doses.

For preclinical PK studies, formulation selection is an important part of the study design. The intravenous formulation is required to be a solution that does not cause significant precipitation or hemolysis upon injection into the blood stream. Common intravenous formulations include vehicles as such as saline and PEG 400-based formulations (PEG = polyethylene glycol).

Oral formulations are highly dependent on the purpose of the oral PK study. Amorphous or crystalline forms of the compound are often formulated in solution or suspension formulations containing components such as PEG 400, 2-hydroxypropyl-β-cyclodextrin (HPBCD), water and Tween 80 in early PK evaluations. These types of early evaluations may provide an optimistic evaluation of the bioavailability as amorphous compounds and solution formulations generally lead to equal or, more likely, higher oral exposure when compared to crystalline compound and suspension formulations. A common formulation used to mimic a tablet in preclinical pharmacokinetic studies is crystalline compound formulated as a methylcellulose based aqueous suspension.

Calculating bioavailability based on IV and PO dosing.

Calculating bioavailability based on IV and PO dosing.	
Given	**Calculations**
Oral Dose – *2 mg/kg* Oral AUC – *20 μg × h/mL* Intravenous Dose – *1 mg/kg* Intravenous AUC - *50 μg × h/mL*	$$F = \frac{20\,/\,2}{50\,/\,1} \times 100 = 20\%$$

6.4   Bioanalysis

Up to the early 1990s, most of the bioanalysis involved liquid chromatography (LC) coupled with ultraviolet light absorption detectors. These methods were not very sensitive and selective, which necessitated both extensive sample clean up (usually liquid-liquid extraction or solid phase extraction) and long chromatographic separation times (>30 min). Alternatively, gas chromatography-mass spectrometry was used for bioanalysis, but this only applies to analytes that can be volatilized, which only represents a small fraction of the analytes. All of this, combined with the poor sensitivity, limited the involvement of DMPK in drug discovery. Things changed dramatically with the introduction of atmospheric pressure ionization (API) mass spectrometry (MS) in the late 1980s. Two types of atmospheric pressure ionization techniques are available: electrospray ionization (ESI) and atmospheric chemical ionization (APCI). Professor John Fenn

---

Study Design Details For Cassette Dosing Pharmacokinetic Studies

Doses

- Low doses prevent interactions that could occur due to co-administration of multiple compounds
- Rat - 0.5 to 2 mg/kg PO / 0.2 to 0.5 mg/kg IV
- Dog - 0.5 to 1 mg/kg PO / 0.2 mg/kg IV

Number of compounds

- Up to 10 compounds

Selection of compounds

- Avoid dosing compounds with same molecular weight
- Check molecular weights of potential metabolites of compounds to avoid bioanalytical assay interference

Biological internal standard

- Preferably of the same chemotype
- A moderate clearance compound allows for easier selection of "winners"
- Dose biological internal standard at 10 times the dose used for cassette studies to assess range of PK linearity

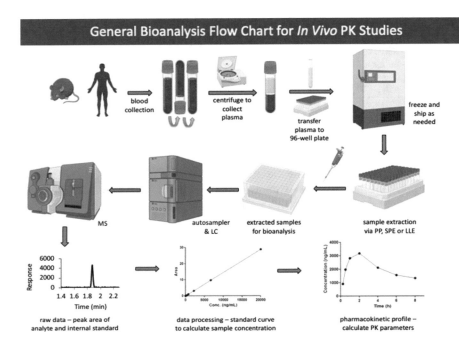

Fig. 6.5 Workflow for bioanalysis of in vivo pharmacokinetic study by LC-MS. (*PP* protein precipitation, *SPE* solid phase extraction; *LLE* liquid-liquid extraction)

was the inventor of ESI and he received the Nobel Prize in 2002. APCI was introduced around the same time as ESI. Both ESI and APCI ionization can easily be interfaced with liquid chromatography equipment and commercial LC-MS equipment for routine use became available in the early 1990s. This dramatically changed the impact of ADME sciences on drug discovery and development. Detection of low concentrations of analytes from both *in vitro* and *in vivo* studies is now routine and data can be generated quickly, which makes it much easier to integrate ADME studies in screening cascades and use the data to influence drug design and optimization.

The workflow for bioanalysis by LC-MS is graphically illustrated in Fig. 6.5 and the key steps are:

1. Sample extraction
2. Chromatographic separation
3. Ionization
4. Mass separation
5. Fragmentation (if MS/MS is employed)
6. Detection

Chromatographic separation has advanced as well. High performance liquid chromatography (HPLC) has been around for many years. Ultra-high performance liquid chromatography (UPLC) was introduced about twenty years ago and combines pumps that operate at much higher pressure with columns having a narrower diameter (≤ 2.1 mm instead of 4.6 mm) and smaller particles (≤ 2 micron instead of 2.5–5 micron). This enables more efficient and rapid mass transfer. The advantages are three-fold: speed, resolution and sensitivity. The down side is higher backpressure, but that can be managed by the higher pressure pumps.

Many analytes have chiral centers. While drugs were marketed as racemic mixtures in the past, stereoisomers can interact differently with the target and can have markedly different potencies. Thus, single stereoisomers are usually pursued these days; they can be synthesized using chirally pure starting materials or the stereoisomers can be separated after synthesis. However, one stereoisomer may convert – either chemically or enzymatically – over time in the other form during *in vitro* or *in vivo* studies. Thus, chiral separation is a necessity and this can be achieved using (1) a chiral stationary phase in the HPLC column or (2) a mobile phase with a chiral reagent. The former is more common. Supercritical fluid chromatography (SFC) is an emerging technique for chiral separation. SFC utilizes supercritical CO_2 as the mobile phase, often mixed with an organic solvent to improve solubility of the analyte and modify the elution strength of the mobile phase. The SFC system must be maintained at a high pressure to ensure that the CO_2 remains in its supercritical state. One of the advantages of SFC is faster analysis time due to lower viscosity and faster mass transfer of the supercritical CO_2. Moreover, CO_2 is a much more environmentally friendly than traditional HPLC solvents such as acetonitrile and methanol.

The most common ionization techniques are electrospray ionization and atmospheric chemical ionization. In electrospray, the liquid is sprayed through a fine needle carrying a high voltage, which imparts a charge to the small liquid droplets. The solvent evaporates and the droplets become smaller and smaller and their charge density increases. Either charged analyte molecules remain or they are expelled from the very small droplets. Subsequently, the charged molecules enter the vacuum of the mass spectrometer. Atmospheric pressure chemical ionization involves a heated nebulizer and a discharge needle carrying a high voltage to generate a "cloud" of reagent ions from the solvent, which can transfer a positive or negative charge to the analyte of interest. Usually, positive ionization mode is used to generate protonated analytes, $[M + H]^+$ ions, because most drugs contain functional group that can easily be pronated. For acids, ionization in the negative ion mode is most suitable and $[M - H]^-$ ions are generated.

The most common type of mass spectrometer is still the triple quadrupole mass spectrometer. They are relatively easy to operate and they are used for virtually all quantitative bioanalysis of small molecules – both preclinical and in the clinic. Triple quadrupole mass spectrometers have two stages of mass spectrometric separation enabling MS/MS. The first quadrupole is set to transmit the molecular weight of the analyte of interest, usually its $[M + H]^+$ ion. Next, this ion enters the second quadrupole where collision with an inert collision gas – usually helium, argon or nitrogen – fragments the $[M + H]^+$ ions into structure characteristic fragment ions. For quantitative purposes, the third quadrupole is usually set to transmit the most abundant fragment ion (while avoiding loss of small molecules, such as H_2O or NH_3, from the $[M + H]^+$ ions because these transitions are less selective). Triple quadrupoles mass spectrometers can easily and quickly switch between different parent ion-fragment ion pairs and this allows for monitoring the analyte of interest and (1) the internal standard (in drug discovery a structurally related compound and in development usually a stable labeled – ^{13}C and or ^2H – analog), (2) one or more metabolites and (3) other analytes of interest. If a single analyte is monitored, it is called selected reaction monitoring (SRM) and if multiple analytes are monitored, it is referred to as multiple reaction monitoring (MRM). Because of the sensitivity and selectivity of LC-MS/MS equipment, sample purification is usually limited to protein precipitation and detection limits of 1 ng/mL and chromatographic run times of a couple of minutes are routine. Using more selective sample purification and sample concentration, detection limits in the low pg/mL can be achieved. The latter is essential when the dose (*in vivo*) or concentration (*in vitro* and *in vivo*) is low; it also enables drug detection using alternative administration routes, such as dermal and inhaled drug delivery, which deliberately results in low systemic drug levels. The use of a triple quadrupole mass spectrometer for determination of the structure of a metabolite is similar as described above, but the third quadrupole is scanned and a complete MS/MS spectrum is obtained. The presence or absence of specific fragment ions can greatly facilitate determination of the structure of the metabolite or, at a minimum, identify the part of the molecule that has been transformed.

High resolution mass spectrometers (HRMS) advanced the field further and they are now the most common instrument used for metabolite identification. HRMS allow determination of the exact mass of the analyte (within about 5 parts per million of the calculated mass) instead of the nominal mass (with unit mass resolution). The reader is reminded that the mass of individual atoms (except carbon) is not an integer; the exact mass and isotopic abundance of atoms most commonly found in drugs are provided in Table 6.10.

If the exact mass of an unknown analyte, *e.g.,* a metabolite, is available, it is feasible to narrow down the number of possible molecular formulas, which facilitates identification of the metabolic biotransformation. The most common instruments capable of high resolution are time-of-flight, orbitrap and Fourier-transform mass spectrometers. These instruments also come with various software packages

Table 6.10 Exact atomic mass and abundance of isotopes of atoms commonly found in drug discovery

Atom	Exact mass (Da)	Isotopic abundance (%)
^{1}H	1.0078	99.985
^{12}C	12.0000	98.9
^{13}C	13.0034	1.1
^{14}N	14.0031	99.6
^{16}O	15.9949	99.8
^{19}F	18.9984	100
^{32}S	31.9721	95.0
^{33}S	32.9715	0.8
^{34}S	33.9679	4.2
^{35}Cl	34.9689	75.5
^{37}Cl	39.9659	24.5
^{79}Br	78.9183	50.5
^{81}Br	80.9163	49.5

that facilitate metabolite detection such as dynamic background subtraction, mass defect filtering, etc.

Thus, LC-MS has advanced the field of ADME tremendously and it is one of the contributing factors that attrition due to poor pharmacokinetics has dropped from about 40% in 1991 to about 10% in 2000 (Kola and Landis 2004). The use of LC-MS has many advantages:

1. High selectivity based on detection of the molecular weight of the analyte, which enables much shorter run times (< 3 minutes is standard and < 1 minute is possible) and differentiation between the parent drug and its metabolites.
2. Improved detection limits, which allows for the routine use of low concentration, *in vitro* ADME studies and the use of low doses for *in vivo* PK studies in drug discovery when quantities of the available drug are limited.

Nevertheless, LC-MS also has its limitation:

1. Not all analytes lend themselves to ionization in either the positive or negative ionization mode. For example, some neutral steroidal compounds have poor ionization efficiencies.
2. The ionization efficiency of analytes can vary greatly and, therefore, it is not possible to obtain the relative abundance of analytes (e.g., the parent compound and its metabolites) by comparing the height of the mass spectrometric signals. Indeed, each analyte needs its own standard curve to allow absolute quantitation. The absence of an authentic standard of metabolites in drug discovery limits its

use in drug discovery and the relative abundance of metabolite signals versus the parent compound has to be interpreted with caution. Parallel use of a UV detector may provide a more quantitative picture because the molar absorptivity varies less between related analytes.

3. It is frequently not possible to come up with the exact structure of the metabolite. For example, mass spectrometric fragmentation patterns usually do not allow you to distinguish isomeric hydroxylated metabolites if the hydroxylation occurred on the same moiety of the parent compound. The structure of some metabolites, such as *N*- or *O*-dealkylation, usually can be established unambiguously. Chemical derivatization and hydrogen-deuterium exchange can provide additional structural information for metabolites (Liu and Hop 2005). Also, the use of structurally related analogs can facilitate interpretation of mass spectrometry data and structural determination of metabolites. Finally, it may be advantageous to isolate the metabolite and perform NMR analysis to get the exact structure. The use of cryogenic probes has greatly improved the sensitivity of NMR analysis – even though it still does not match that of LC-MS.

An additional technical advancement was provided by the invention of matrix-assisted laser desorption/ionization (MALDI) by Professor Franz Hillenkamp and Professor Michael Karas in 1985. Knowing the tissue concentration can advance interpretation of efficacy and toxicology studies. Even though it is possible to determine the concentration of analytes in tissues by excising and homogenizing the tissue and then performing LC-MS/MS, the concentration in substructures of the organ is frequently lost. MALDI imaging (Caprioli et al. 1997) allows you to do exactly that. The organ of interest is isolated, frozen and sliced. A very thin tissue slice is sprayed with a UV-absorbing matrix such as dihydroxy benzoic acid. After evaporation of the solvent, the tissue is transferred to the vacuum of the mass spectrometer and a laser is scanned in discrete steps across the tissue slice. The matrix ions are ionized and they, subsequently, transfer a positive or negative charge to the analyte of interest. The most common mass analyzers for MALDI imaging are time-of-flight and Fourier-transform mass spectrometers. Detection of both the parent compound and its metabolites is possible with a spatial resolution of up to 25 μm. There are various other valuable imaging techniques, such as quantitative whole-body autoradiography and PET imaging, but they require – in contrast to MALDI imaging – radiolabeled drugs, which are usually not available in drug discovery.

Further technical details of sample preparation, chromatographic separation and mass spectrometric detection, including the advantages and disadvantages of various approaches, are provided in DMPK Quick Guide.

Applications LC-MS/MS is the usual bioanalytical endpoint for most quantitative *in vitro* ADME studies such as metabolic stability in microsomes, cytosol or hepatocytes, plasma protein binding or binding in other matrices, blood to plasma partitioning, competitive and time-dependent CYP inhibition, CYP induction, permeability in MDCK cells, Caco-2 cells or PAMPA, and transport in cells that overexpress uptake or efflux transporters. Generally, the experimental matrices are relatively clean and sample preparation is usually limited to protein precipitation. Rapid LC column switching or multiplexing and/or sample pooling is used to enhance throughput. The approach for determination of the drug concentration in samples from either preclinical or clinical *in vivo* studies is generally similar, but sample preparation and other experimental variables may be more rigorous to (1) improve the detection limit, (2) eliminate interference, or (3) meet strict regulatory method validation guidelines for Good Laboratory Practice (GLP) toxicity studies or clinical studies. Sample pooling or cassette dosing can be employed for preclinical studies. Cassette dosing involves administration of multiple compounds simultaneously to an animal. To avoid or assess drug-drug interaction between these compounds, the doses are kept low and/or a control compound with known pharmacokinetics is included. Finally, the degree of method development employed is always 'fit for purpose'. The amount of method optimization is minimal for most drug discovery studies, but may be more rigorous for data included in a regulatory submission. GLP bioanalysis for toxicity studies and clinical bioanalysis requires much more rigorous method development and validation and is described in detail in FDA and EMA guidance documents (Food and Drug Administration 2018; European Medicines Agency 2011).

> Microsampling (< 50 µL) has become more popular for both preclinical and clinical *in vivo* studies. Microsampling is less invasive and painful than traditional sampling methods in the clinic and can be applied to pediatric patients. Equally, it can reduce distress in animals, in particular in rodents, and it also avoids having to use a separate satellite group of rodents for toxicokinetics in toxicology studies. With more and more sensitive LC-MS equipment, the reduced amount of material – either blood or plasma – should not be a challenge.

The process for the use of LC-MS/MS for metabolite identification is described above. The purpose for metabolite identification is diverse and includes:

1. Determination of the major metabolic liability in the molecule to facilitate identification of a molecule with more favorable pharmacokinetic properties.
2. Determination of the enzymes involved in metabolism of a compound.
3. Determination if the *in vitro* metabolic pathways in human liver microsomes, cytosol or hepatocytes is similar to that observed in preclinical species; this assessment will influence the selection of the species used in preclinical toxicity studies.

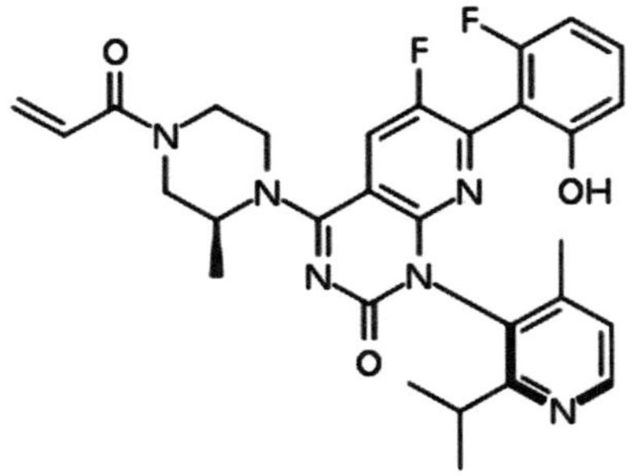

Fig. 6.6 Molecular
structure of sotorasib, a
RAS G12C inhibitor

4. Determination of the metabolites present in human plasma from clinical studies
   and assessment if the toxicology species were exposed to the same amount or
   more to provide coverage; if not, dedicated toxicology studies with metabolites
   may be required.

Another interesting application of LC-MS/MS is it use for the detection of covalent adducts. Covalent inhibitors have become more popular – initially for life-
threatening indications such as in oncology, but now also for non-life-threatening
use. The approach is similar to the ubiquitous use of LC-MS/MS in proteomics.
First, the proteins are subjected to enzymatic digestion and the resulting peptides
are analyzed by LC-MS/MS. In this case, the target protein of interest is known
and you look for a peptide that has been covalently modified. The fragmentation
pattern of that peptide identifies the covalently modified amino acid, e.g. Amgen's
sotorasib covalently modifies the cysteine residue that is mutated in RAS G12C
(Fig. 6.6).

6.5   Supplemental Tables

Cofactors are key ingredients needed to activate many drug metabolizing enzymes.
The cofactors are used in excess of what is needed to assure that they do not become
a rate limiting compound. NADPH can be used in the reduced formed or in a regen-
erating system with $NADP^+$ and glucose 6-phosphate and glucose 6-phosphatase.
While NADPH is more expensive, the advantage is that it removes the need for a
pre-incubation and reduces the number of reagents that need to be added to the
incubation.

Table 6.S.1 The names and chemical structures of cofactors used by drug metabolizing enzymes

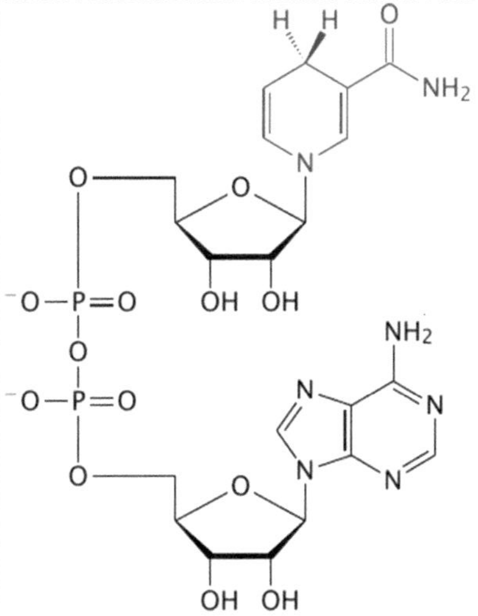

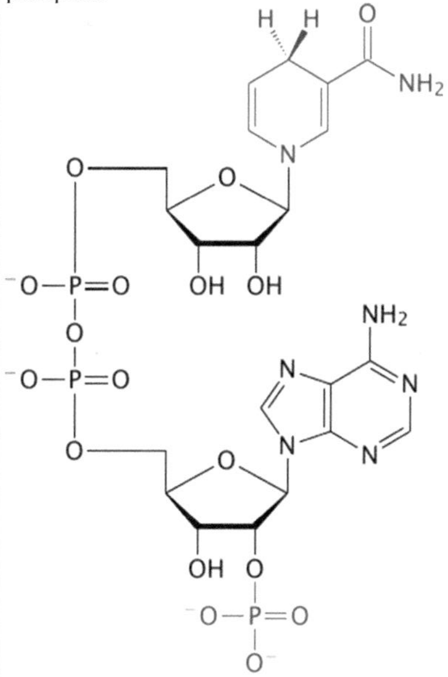

Cofactor	Structure and full name	Cofactor	Structure and full name
NADH	Reduced nicotinamide adenine dinucleotide	NADPH	Reduced nicotinamide adenine dinucleotide phosphate

| UDPGA | Uridine diphosphate glucuronic acid 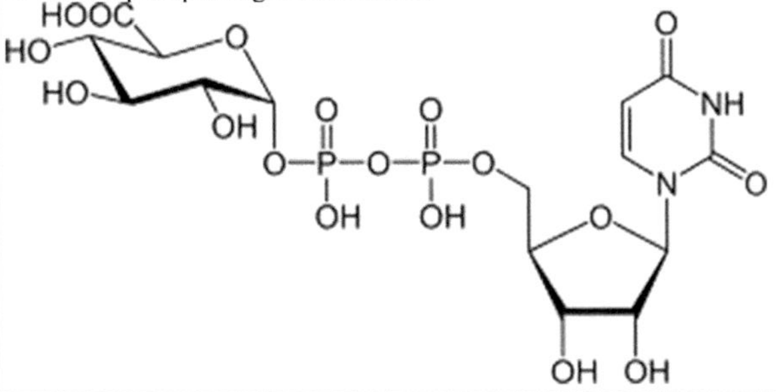 | SAM | S-Adenosyl methionine 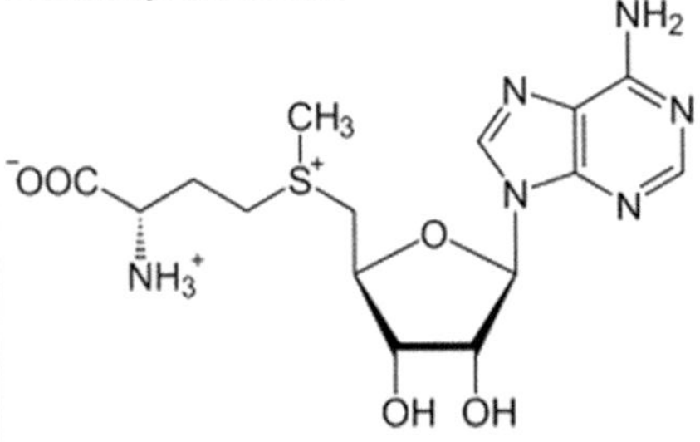 |
| Acetyl CoA | Acetyl coenzyme A 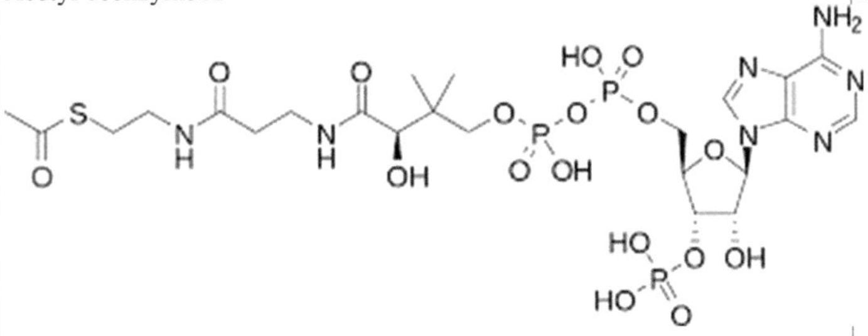 | PAPS | 3'-Phosphoadenosine-5'-phosphosulfate 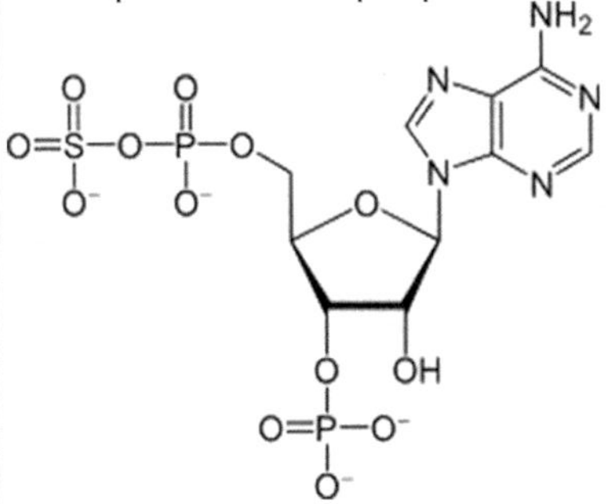 |

Table 6.S.2 Incubation conditions for metabolic stability assays using cells, tissue fractions, or recombinant enzymes

Cells	<u>Hepatocytes:</u> A more complete system than LM and more representative of a physiological system since it includes cellular barriers and the presence of transporters
	More challenging to work with compared to tissue fractions. Cell viability needs to be considered (species differences observed)
	Typical cell density 0.5 x 10⁶ cell/mL; incubate at 37 °C in 5% CO_2 with saturating humidity
	Suspended cryopreserved hepatocytes are the most common tools to examine general metabolic stability. They closely resemble the initial expression of the enzymes. However, they are vulnerable and undergo changes during the incubation
	Plated hepatocytes with a high density, allowing for cell-to-cell contact, may result in increased cell viability; the expression of DMEs are typically lower, unless they are induced or co-cultured. New advances with co-cultures allow the cell to maintain cell viability plus an appropriate expression of DMEs. Plated hepatocytes tend to be more expensive and are, therefore, used for compounds that are further along the development process when a more robust analysis of metabolic stability is required (Bonn et al. 2016)
	<u>Enterocytes:</u> now commercially available (Ho et al. 2017)
Tissue fractions	<u>Liver microsomes (LM)</u>
	LM include many different types of DME including both Phase I and II enzymes. Since cofactors are present in the cytosolic fraction, LM have to be fortified with the necessary cofactors in the incubations. Two major DMEs that are present in LM are CYP and UGT, which need NADPH and UDPGA, respectively. Typically, CYP provides a good correlation to *in vivo* data but UGT reactions, like many others, are under-estimated. UGT is present on the luminal side of the endoplasmic reticulum (ER; converts to microsomes); therefore, pore-forming peptides (such as alamethicin; Fisher et al. 2000) or detergents are often needed to provide access to this enzyme. Note that many CYP enzymes are typically inhibited by detergents
	Improved kinetics are calculated based on lower enzyme concentrations, but on the other hand, a high concentration of enzymes provides higher turnover, leading to a better ability to define stability regions
	The sex of the tissue should also be considered. For example, in the case of rats, stark sex-dependent differences are observed
	<u>Cytosol:</u> Contains a large pool of DMEs such as aldehyde oxidases, hydrolases, and *N*-acetyl transferases. Most of these DMEs do not require further fortifications of cofactors, but one exception is *N*-acetyl transferase, which requires acetyl-CoA
	<u>Lysosomes:</u> This is important for proteolysis. Studies with S9 fractions have shown that lowering the pH allows for a better lysosomal activity
Recombinant enzymes	Many commercially recombinant enzymes can be used; CYP, UGT, and others

Table 6.S.3 Considerations for the buffer, solvent, and test article in metabolic stability assays

Buffer	The most common buffer is potassium phosphate (KPi; the "i" is for "inorganic") at usually 50–100 mM with pH adjusted to 7.4 (intercellular pH)
	Other types of buffers can be used, but be aware that the buffer does not inhibit or activate the targeted DME. Activation of enzymes by ions has been reported. For example, CYP enzymes can be activated by the magnesium ion at 10 mM (Schrag and Wienkers 2000)
	A commonly used incubation buffer for hepatocytes is Dulbecco's modified eagle medium (DMEM)
Organic solvents	Organic solvents should be kept at as minimum a concentration as possible. This is typically less than 1%, and for DMSO the concentration should be no more than 0.1%
	Organic solvents are used to transfer test articles to the incubation. The compounds are typically soluble in organic solvents and can be kept in long-term storage
	Stock solutions of test compounds are usually made with DMSO and are typically 1000–10,000 more concentrated than the incubation concentration
	It is advisable that dilutions be make in buffer prior to addition to the incubation mixture.
	Other possible solvents include acetonitrile and methanol
	Relative to water, acetonitrile and methanol have less inhibitory properties. DMSO is very inhibitory but at the same time the most useful due to its high boiling point and solvation of insoluble compounds (González-Pérez et al. 2012)
Compound concentration [S]	The compound should be incubated at physiological relevant concentrations
	Test compound concentrations are usually 1 µM or lower. Historically, the low sensitivity of detection methods required a high concentration; however, this is no longer the case and lower concentrations can be used
	Compund concentrations less than the K_m result in zero order kinetics (rate is independent of [S])
	Most DMEs have K_m values higher than 1 µM, but this is not always true. Saturation kinetics is observed when [S] reaches K_m

Table 6.S.4 Considerations for the automation of metabolic stability assays

Plates/tubes	The choice of plates is an important aspect for a couple reason. First, compound adhesion to the plate could lead to data that is mistakenly interpreted as a liability in stability. Adhesion to the plate is compound dependent and needs to be examined experimentally. Testing the compound in buffer in the absence of LM is a good control. Second, experiments are performed in plates that allow for several incubations to be performed simultaneously on a smaller scale. 96-well plates are often used, but higher throughput plates with 384 wells and above can also be used. Considerations include the well size, transfer volumes, and ability to mix
Volume transfers	The instrument must be able to accurately transfer the range of volumes required to complete the assay
Time for waiting	The amount of time that each plate waits on an instrument platform should be minimized to avoid enzyme inactivation before the start of the reaction. This is especially true when the incubation solution is at 37 °C

Table 6.S.5 Sequence of addition, incubation time, replicates, and assay controls for metabolic stability assays

Sequence of addition	If the compound is a substrate of CYP or UGT only, the cofactor can be added in the last step. This allows for equilibrium to be reached between the substrate and the potential DME
	However, this information is not always known. In addition, other types of reactions could occur, such as hydrolysis, which requires only water to catalyze the reaction. In light of this, the test compounds can be added in the last step to minimize unwanted reactions prior to starting the clock for recording reaction time
Incubation time	For LM, incubations can last up to 60 min. Longer incubation times may lead to non-linear kinetics and a slower rate. Part of the inactivation by CYP in this type of reaction is due to the ROS formed during the oxidation process
	For cryopreserved hepatocyte suspensions, incubations can last up to 3 hours
Replicates	N = 1 or 3, depending on whether this is a routine screening or a more definitive study, respectively
	Studies with fewer timepoints usually include more replicates (N = 2 or 3) than studies with more timepoints (N = 1)
Controls	A robust analysis requires the use of control compounds in order to compare between multiple runs. Controls should cover a range of stability from very stable to labile. A cocktail of controls allows for testing several types of enzymes
	One such control could be the examination of test article stability in the absence of cofactor

Table 6.S.6 Quenching, sample preparation, and bioanalysis of metabolic stability assays

Quenching	The quenching solution is acetonitrile with 0.1% formic acid and an internal standard
Internal standard (IS)	An IS is used to check compound recovery, the analytical process, and MS detection
	If possible, it is best to use an IS with similar properties to the analyte
Sample preparation	Samples are centrifuged at 2000 g for 20 min to precipitate the protein. The supernatants are removed and diluted with a six-fold volume of water to dilute the organic solvent
	Several compounds can be tested in one incubation through the use of cassetting techniques
Bioanalysis	Samples are analyzed by LC-MS for disappearance of parent compound and formation of metabolite(s). Typically, MRM in positive ion mode is used. High resolution MS has opened the door to performing studies without MRM optimization, and therefore MS conditions do not need to be optimized for each compound

Table 6.S.7 Predicted hepatic clearance (CL_h) calculted from half-life in liver microsomes

Parameters	Calculations	Units
Half-life ($t_{1/2}$)		Min
	$\dfrac{[0.693}{K}$ $(\ln_2 = 0.693)$	
CL_{int}	Slope x (-2.303) x (mL/mg LM) x (mg LM/g liver) x (g liver/ kg)	Mg/min/kg
CL_h	$(Q_h * fu_{blood} * CL_{int} / fu_{LM}) / (Q_h + (fu_{blood} * CL_{int}/fu_{LM}))$	Mg/min/kg

The calculated parameters are half-life ($t_{1/2}$), intrinsic clearance (CL_{int}), and CL_h. The inputs are liver blood flow (Q_h) and fraction unbound in blood (fu_{blood}) and in liver microsomes (fu_{LM}).

Table 6.S.8 List of common primary Phase I and Phase II biotransformation pathways and the corresponding elemental composition, accurate m/z, and mass defect changes

Metabolic reaction	Description	Elemental composition change	m/z shift	Mass defect change (mDa)
R-X-C$_2$H$_5$ → R-X-H (X = N, O, S)	Deethylation	- C$_2$H$_4$	−28.0313	−31.3
RR'-CH-OH → R-CHO	Alcohols to aldehyde/ketone	- H$_2$	−2.0157	−15.7
R-CH$_2$-NH$_2$ → R-CH$_2$-OH	Oxidative deamination to alcohol	- NH + O	0.9840	−16.0
R-CO-R' → R-CHOH-R'	Reduction	+ H$_2$	2.0157	15.7
R-CH$_2$-R' → R-C(O)-R'	Oxidation (methylene to ketone)	- H$_2$ + O	13.9793	−20.7
R-XH → R-X-CH$_3$ (X = N, O, S)	N, O, S methylation	+ CH$_2$	14.0157	15.7
R-H → R-OH	Hydroxylation	+ O	15.9949	−5.10
R-NH-R' → R-NOH-R' RR'R"N → RR'R"NO	2^0 & 3^0 amine to hydroxylamine/N-oxide	+ O	15.9949	−5.10
R-S-R' → R-SO-R' R-SO-R' → R-SO$_2$-R'	Thioether to sulfoxide Sulfoxide to sulfone	+ O	15.9949	−5.10
R-CH=CH-R' → R-CH(OH)-CH(OH)-R'	Dihydroxylation	+ H$_2$O$_2$	34.0055	5.50
R-NH$_2$ → R-NHCOCH$_3$	Acetylation	+ C$_2$H$_2$O	42.0106	10.6
R-COOH → R-CONHCH$_2$COOH	Glycine conjugation	+ C$_2$H$_3$NO	57.0215	21.5
R-OH → R-OSO$_3$H	Sulfonation	+ SO$_3$	79.9568	−43.2
R-COOH → R-CONH-CH$_2$CH$_2$SO$_3$H	Taurine conjugation	+ C$_2$H$_5$NO$_2$S	107.0041	4.10
R$_3$-CH → R3-C-SCH$_2$CH(NH$_2$)CO$_2$H	S-cysteine conjugation	+ C$_3$H$_5$NO$_2$S	119.0041	4.10
R$_3$-CH → R$_3$-C-SCH$_2$CH(NHCOCH$_3$)-CO$_2$H	N-acetylcysteine conjugation	+ C$_5$H$_7$NO$_3$S	161.0147	14.7
R-OH → R-O-C$_6$H$_{11}$O$_5$	Glucosidation	+ C$_6$H$_{10}$O$_5$	162.0528	52.8
R-OH → R-O-C$_6$H$_9$O$_6$	Glucuronidation	+ C$_6$H$_8$O$_6$	176.0321	32.1
+ GSH - 2H	GSH conjugation	+ C$_{10}$H$_{15}$N$_3$O$_6$S	305.0682	68.2
+ GSH	GSH conj.	+ C$_{10}$H$_{17}$N$_3$O$_6$S	307.0838	83.8
+ GSH + O - 2H	Oxidation + GSH conj.	+ C$_{10}$H$_{15}$N$_3$O$_7$S	321.0631	63.1
Epoxidation + GSH	Epoxidation + GSH conj.	+ C$_{10}$H$_{17}$N$_3$O$_7$S	323.0787	78.8

References

Bonn B, Svanberg P, Janefeldt A, Hultman I, Grime K (2016) Determination of human hepatocyte intrinsic clearance for slowly metabolized compounds: comparison of a primary hepatocyte/stromal cell co-culture with plated primary hepatocytes and HepaRG. Drug Metab Dispos 44(4):527–533. https://doi.org/10.1124/dmd.115.067769

Caprioli RM, Farmer TB, Gile J (1997) Molecular imaging of biological samples: localization of peptides and proteins using MALDI-TOF MS. Anal Chem 69(23):4751–4760

Cerny MA (2016) Prevalence of non–cytochrome P450–mediated metabolism in Food and Drug Administration–approved oral and intravenous drugs: 2006–2015. Drug Metab Dispos 44(8):1246–1252. https://doi.org/10.1124/dmd.116.070763

Chen Y-C, Kenny JR, Wright M, Hop CECA, Yan Z (2018) Improving confidence in the determination of free fraction for highly bound drugs using bi-directional equilibrium dialysis. J Pharm Sci 108(3):1296–1302. https://doi.org/10.1016/j.xphs.2018.10.011

Choo EF, Salphati L (2018) Leveraging humanized animal models to understand human drug disposition: opportunities, challenges, and future directions. Clin Pharmacol Ther 103(2):188–192. https://doi.org/10.1002/cpt.908

Dash RP, Veeravalli V, Thomas JA, Rosenfeld C, Mehta N, Srinivas NR (2021) Whole blood or plasma: what is the ideal matrix for pharmacokinetic-driven drug candidate selection? Future Med Chem 13(2):157–171. https://doi.org/10.4155/fmc-2020-0187

Day SH, Mao A, White R, Schulz-Utermoehl T, Miller R, Beconi MG (2005) A semi-automated method for measuring the potential for protein covalent binding in drug discovery. J Pharmacol Toxicol Methods 52(2):278–285. https://doi.org/10.1016/j.vascn.2004.11.006

Evans DC, Watt AP, Nicoll-Griffith DA, Baillie TA (2004) Drug-protein adducts: an industry perspective on minimizing the potential for drug bioactivation in drug discovery and development. Chem Res Toxicol 17(1):3–16

European Medicines Agency (2011) https://www.ema.europa.eu/en/documents/scientific-guideline/guideline-bioanalytical-method-validation_en.pdf

Fisher MB, Campanale K, Ackermann BL, VandenBranden M, Wrighton SA (2000) In vitro glucuronidation using human liver microsomes and the pore-forming peptide alamethicin. Drug Metab Dispos 28(5):560–566

Fitch WL, Khojasteh C, Aliagas I, Johnson K (2018) Using LC retention times in organic structure determination: drug metabolite identification. Drug Metabolism Lett 12(2):93–100. https://doi.org/10.2174/1872312812666180802093347

Food and Drug Administration (2018) Guidance for industry: bioanalytical method validation. US Department of Health and Human Services, FDA, Center for Drug Evaluation and Research and Center for Veterinary Medicine, Rockville, MD. https://www.fda.gov/media/70858/download

Gan J, Harper TW, Hsueh MM, Qu Q, Humphreys WG (2005) Dansyl glutathione as a trapping agent for the quantitative estimation and identification of reactive metabolites. Chem Res Toxicol 18(5):896–903. https://doi.org/10.1021/tx0496791

Goetz GH, Philippe L, Shapiro MJ (2014) EPSA: a novel supercritical fluid chromatography technique enabling the design of permeable cyclic peptides. ACS Med Chem Lett 5(10):1167–1172. https://doi.org/10.1021/ml500239m

González-Pérez V, Connolly EA, Bridges AS (2012) Impact of organic solvents on cytochrome P450 probe reactions: filling the gap with (s)-warfarin and midazolam hydroxylation. Drug Metab Dispos 40(11):2136–2142. https://doi.org/10.1124/dmd.112.047134

Halladay JS, Wong S, Khojasteh SC, Grepper S (2012) An 'all-inclusive' 96-well cytochrome P450 induction method: measuring enzyme activity, mRNA levels, protein levels, and cytotoxicity from one well using cryopreserved human hepatocytes. J Pharmacol Toxicol 66(3):270–275. https://doi.org/10.1016/j.vascn.2012.07.004

Hewitt NJ, Lecluyse EL, Ferguson SS (2008) Induction of hepatic cytochrome P450 enzymes: methods, mechanisms, recommendations, and in vitro–in vivo correlations. Xenobiotica 37(10–11):1196–1224. https://doi.org/10.1080/00498250701534893

Ho M-CD, Ring N, Amaral K, Doshi U, Li A (2017) Human enterocytes as an in vitro model for the evaluation of intestinal drug metabolism: characterization of drug metabolizing enzyme activities of cryopreserved human enterocytes from twenty four donors. Drug Metab Dispos 45(6):dmd.116.074377. https://doi.org/10.1124/dmd.116.074377

Kenny JR, Ramsden D, Buckley DB et al (2018) Considerations from the IQ induction working group in response to drug-drug interaction guidances from regulatory agencies: focus on CYP3A4 mRNA in vitro response thresholds, variability, and clinical relevance. Drug Metab Dispos 46(9):dmd.118.081927. https://doi.org/10.1124/dmd.118.081927

Khojasteh SC, Prabhu S, Kenny JR, Halladay JS, Lu AYH (2011) Chemical inhibitors of cytochrome P450 isoforms in human liver microsomes: a re-evaluation of P450 isoform selectivity. Eur J Drug Metab Ph 36(1):1–16. https://doi.org/10.1007/s13318-011-0024-2

Kola I, Landis J (2004) Can the pharmaceutical industry reduce attrition rates? Nature Rev Drug Discov 3(8):711–715

Kosaka M, Zhang D, Wong S, Yan Z (2020) NADPH-independent inactivation of CYP2B6 and NADPH-dependent inactivation of CYP3A4/5 by PBD: potential implication for assessing covalent modulators for time-dependent inhibition. Drug Metab Dispos 48(8):655–661. https://doi.org/10.1124/dmd.120.090878. Epub 2020 Jun 1

Leung C, Kenny JR, Hop CECA, Yan Z (2020) Strategy for determining the free fraction of labile covalent modulators in plasma using equilibrium dialysis. J Pharm Sci 9(10):3181–3189. https://doi.org/10.1016/j.xphs.2020.06.029. Epub 2020 Jul 12

Liu D, Hop CECA (2005) Strategies for characterization of drug metabolites using liquid chromatography-tandem mass spectrometry in conjunction with chemical derivatization and on-line H/D exchange approaches. J Pharm Biomed Anal 37(1):1–18

Luco JM, Salinas AP, Torriero AAJ, Vázquez RN, Raba J, Marchevsky E (2003) Immobilized artificial membrane chromatography: quantitative structure-retention relationships of structurally diverse drugs. J Chem Inf Comput Sci 43(6):2129–2136. https://doi.org/10.1021/ci034123p

Mao J, Mohutsky MA, Harrelson JP, Wrighton SA, Hall SD (2012) Predictions of cytochrome P450-mediated drug-drug interactions using cryopreserved human hepatocytes: comparison of plasma and protein-free media incubation conditions. Drug Metab Dispos 40(4):706–716. https://doi.org/10.1124/dmd.111.043158

Mukadam S, Tay S, Tran D et al (2012) Evaluation of time-dependent cytochrome P450 inhibition in a high-throughput, automated assay: introducing a novel area under the curve shift approach. Drug Metab Lett 6(1):43–53. https://doi.org/10.2174/187231212800229309

Romagnoli N, Al-Qudah KM, Armorini S, Lambertini C, Zaghini A, Spadari A, Roncada P (2017) Pharmacokinetic profile and partitioning in red blood cells of romifidine after single intravenous administration in the horse. Vet Med Sci 3(4):187–197. https://doi.org/10.1002/vms3.70

Obach RS, Kalgutkar AS, Soglia JR, Zhao SX (2008) Can in vitro metabolism-dependent covalent binding data in liver microsomes distinguish hepatotoxic from nonhepatotoxic drugs? An analysis of 18 drugs with consideration of intrinsic clearance and daily dose. Chem Res Toxicol 21(9):1814–1822. https://doi.org/10.1021/tx800161s

Sambuy Y, Angelis ID, Ranaldi G, Scarino ML, Stammati A, Zucco F (2005) The Caco-2 cell line as a model of the intestinal barrier: influence of cell and culture-related factors on Caco-2 cell functional characteristics. Cell Biol Toxicol 21(1):1–26. https://doi.org/10.1007/s10565-005-0085-6

Schadt S, Simon S, Kustermann S et al (2015) Minimizing DILI risk in drug discovery - a screening tool for drug candidates. Toxicol In Vitro 25:429–437

Schrag ML, Wienkers LC (2000) Topological alteration of the CYP3A4 active site by the divalent cation mg(2+). Drug Metab Dispos 28(10):1198–1201

Soglia JR, Contillo LG, Kalgutkar AS, Zhao S, Hop CE, Boyd JG, Cole MJ (2006) A semiquantitative method for the determination of reactive metabolite conjugate levels in vitro utilizing liquid chromatography-tandem mass spectrometry and novel quaternary ammonium glutathione analogues. Chem Res Toxicol 19(3):480–490. https://doi.org/10.1021/tx050303c

Yan Z, Caldwell GW (2004) Stable-isotope trapping and high-throughput screenings of reactive metabolites using the isotope MS signature. Anal Chem 76(23):6835–6847. https://doi.org/10.1021/ac040159k

Wang C, Williams NS (2013) A mass balance approach for calculation of recovery and binding enables the use of ultrafiltration as a rapid method for measurement of plasma protein binding for even highly lipophilic compounds. J Pharmaceut Biomed 75:112–117. https://doi.org/10.1016/j.jpba.2012.11.018

Waters NJ, Jones R, Williams G, Sohal B (2008) Validation of a rapid equilibrium dialysis approach for the measurement of plasma protein binding. J Pharm Sci 97(10):4586–4595. https://doi.org/10.1002/jps.21317

Wei C, Chupak LS, Philip T et al (2013) Screening and characterization of reactive compounds with in vitro peptide-trapping and liquid chromatography/high-resolution accurate mass spectrometry. J Biomol Screen 19(2):297–307. https://doi.org/10.1177/1087057113492852

Wong H, Chen JZ, Chou B, Halladay JS, Kenny JR, La H, Marsters JC Jr, Plise E, Rudewicz PJ, Robarge K, Shin Y, Wong S, Zhang C, Khojasteh SC (2009) Preclinical assessment of the absorption, distribution, metabolism and excretion of GDC-0449 (2-chloro-N-(4-chloro-3-(pyridin-2-yl)phenyl)-4-(methylsulfonyl)benzamide), an orally bioavailable systemic hedgehog signalling pathway inhibitor. Xenobiotica 39(11):850–861. https://doi.org/10.3109/00498250903180289

Zientek MA, Youdim K (2015) Reaction phenotyping: advances in the experimental strategies used to characterize the contribution of drug-metabolizing enzymes. Drug Metab Dispos 43(1):163–181. https://doi.org/10.1124/dmd.114.058750

Chapter 7
Regulatory Documents for IND to Support FIH

Contents

Abstract This chapter is used as a reference for provided various resources as it comes to regulatory authorities. This includes the counties, codes of US federal regulations, IND sections plus various modules and notable guidance for industry by FDA.

Keywords Regulatory authorities · Regulatory guidance

Abbreviations

AIFA	Italian Medicines Agency
ANSM	French National Agency for Medicines and Health Products Safety
ANVISA	National Health Surveillance Agency
CFDA	China Food and Drug Administration
COFEPRIS	Federal Commission for the Protection against Sanitary Risks
CRF	Code of Federal Regulations
CTD	Common Technical Document for the Registration of Pharmaceuticals for Human Use
DG-SANCO	European Commission - Directorate General for Health and Consumers
EMA	European Medicines Agency
FDA	Food and Drug Administration

© Springer Nature Switzerland AG 2022   217
S. C. Khojasteh et al., *Discovery DMPK Quick Guide*,
https://doi.org/10.1007/978-3-031-10691-0_7

GLP	Good Laboratory Practices
HAS	Health Sciences Authority Singapore
HPFB-HC	Health Products and Food Branch, Health Canada
HPRA	Health Product Regulatory Authority
MCC	Medicines Control Council, Department of Health
MEB	Medicines Evaluation Board
Medsafe	New Zealand Medicines and Medical Devices Safety
MFDS	Ministry of Food and Drug Safety
MGLW	Ministry of Health, Labour and Welfare
MHRA	Medicines and Healthcare Products Regulatory Agency
NAFDAC	National Agency for Food Drug Administration and Control
PEI	Paul-Ehrlich-Institute
PMDA	Pharmaceuticals and Medical Devices Agency
TGA	Therapeutic Goods Administration

7.1 Regulatory Authorities in Different Countries

Table 7.1 Regulatory authorities in different countries

Continent	Country	Name (Abbreviation)
Africa	Nigeria South Africa	National Agency for Food Drug Administration and Control (**NAFDAC**) Medicines Control Council, Department of Health (**MCC**)
Asia	China Japan Japan S. Korea Singapore	China Food and Drug Administration (**CFDA**) Pharmaceuticals and Medical Devices Agency (**PMDA**) Ministry of Health, Labour and Welfare (**MGLW**) Ministry of Food and Drug Safety (**MFDS**) Health Sciences Authority Singapore (**HAS**)
Europe	Collective France Germany Ireland Italy Netherlands Switzerland UK	European Commission - Directorate General for Health and Consumers (**DG-SANCO**) European Medicines Agency (**EMA**) French National Agency for Medicines and Health Products Safety (**ANSM**) Paul-Ehrlich-Institute (**PEI**) Health Product Regulatory Authority (**HPRA**) Italian Medicines Agency (**AIFA**) Medicines Evaluation Board (**MEB**) Swissmedic Medicines and Healthcare Products Regulatory Agency (**MHRA**)
North America	Canada Mexico USA	Health Products and Food Branch, Health Canada (**HPFB-HC**) Federal Commission for the Protection against Sanitary Risks (**COFEPRIS**) Food and Drug Administration (**FDA**)
Oceania	Australia New Zealand	Therapeutic Goods Administration (**TGA**) New Zealand Medicines and Medical Devices Safety (**Medsafe**)
South America	Brazil	National Health Surveillance Agency (**ANVISA**)

Table 7.2 Notable section Title 21 is the portion of the Code of Federal Regulations that governs food and drugs within the United States for the Food and Drug Administration

Part	Name
11	Electronic records and electronic signature related
50	Protection of human subjects in clinical trials
54	Financial Disclosure by Clinical Investigators [2]
56	Institutional Review Boards that oversee clinical trials
58	Good Laboratory Practices (GLP) for nonclinical studies
201	Drug Labeling
312	Investigational New Drug Application
314	INDA and NDA Applications for FDA Approval to Market a New Drug
316	Orphan Drugs

7.2 Code of Federal Regulations (US)

The Code of Federal Regulations (CFR) is the codification of the general and permanent rules and regulations. The CFR is divided into 50 titles that represent broad areas subject to federal regulation. Title 21 is the portion of the CFR that governs food and drugs within the United States for the Food and Drug Administration (FDA) (Table 7.2).

7.3 IND Sections

There are four main pieces of information that ADME scientists contribute to INDs:

1. Exposures that achieve efficacy in preclinical species
2. Exposures that achieve safety and toxicity in preclinical species
3. ADME properties from preclinical species
4. Prediction of human exposure and risk assessment

The guidance for industry can be found here: https://www.fda.gov/media/71628/download.

Excerpt from This Document This is one in a series of guidances that provide recommendations for applicants preparing the Common Technical Document for the Registration of Pharmaceuticals for Human Use (CTD) for submission to the U.S. Food and Drug Administration (FDA). This guidance presents the agreed upon common format for the preparation of a well-structured Safety section of the CTD for applications that will be submitted to regulatory authorities. A common format for the technical documentation will significantly reduce the time and resources used to compile applications for registration of human pharmaceuticals and will ease the preparation of electronic submissions. Regulatory reviews and communication with the applicant will be facilitated by a standard document of common elements. In addition, exchange of regulatory information among regulatory authorities will be simplified.

The CTD should be organized into five modules. Module 1 is region specific. Modules 2, 3, 4, and 5 are intended to be common for all regions. Conformance with the CTD guidances should help ensure that these four modules are provided in a format acceptable to the regulatory authorities (see the figure and overall outline on the following pages).

The CTD should be organized according to the following general outline.

Module 1: Administrative Information and Prescribing Information.

  1.1. Table of Contents of the Submission Including Module 1.
  1.2. Documents Specific to Each Region (for example, application forms, prescribing information).

Module 2: Common Technical Document Summaries.

  2.1 CTD Table of Contents.
  2.2 CTD Introduction.
  2.3 Quality Overall Summary.
  2.4 Nonclinical Overview.
  2.5 Clinical Overview.
  2.6 Nonclinical   Written   and   Tabulated   Summaries   Pharmacology Pharmacokinetics Toxicology 2.7 Clinical Summary Biopharmaceutics and Associated Analytical Methods Clinical Pharmacology Studies Clinical Efficacy Clinical Safety Synopses of Individual Studies.

Module 3: Quality.

  3.1 Module 3 Table of Contents.
  3.2 Body of Data.
  3.3 Literature References.

Module 4: Nonclinical Study Reports.

  4.1 Module 4 Table of Contents.
  4.2 Study Reports.
  4.3 Literature References.

Module 5: Clinical Study Reports.

  5.1 Module 5 Table of Contents.
  5.2 Tabular Listing of All Clinical Studies.
  5.3 Clinical Study Reports.
  5.4 Literature References.

4.2 STUDY REPORTS

The study reports should be presented in the following order:

4.2.1 Pharmacology.

4.2.1.1 Primary Pharmacodynamics.
4.2.1.2 Secondary Pharmacodynamics.
4.2.1.3 Safety Pharmacology.
4.2.1.4 Pharmacodynamic Drug Interactions.

4.2.2 Pharmacokinetics.

4.2.2.1 Analytical Methods and Validation Reports (if separate reports are available).
4.2.2.2 Absorption.
4.2.2.3 Distribution.
4.2.2.4 Metabolism.
4.2.2.5 Excretion.
4.2.2.6 Pharmacokinetic Drug Interactions (nonclinical).
4.2.2.7 Other Pharmacokinetic Studies.

7.4   Notable FDA Guidance for Industry

Table 7.3 Notable FDA guidance for industry

Name	Date
S11 Nonclinical Safety Testing In Support of Development of Pediatric Pharmaceuticals	May 2021
Safety Testing of Drug Metabolites	Mar 2020
Clinical Drug Interaction Studies — Cytochrome P450 Enzyme- and Transporter-Mediated Drug Interactions Guidance for Industry	Jan 2020
In Vitro Drug Interaction Studies — Cytochrome P450 Enzyme- and Transporter-Mediated Drug Interactions Guidance for Industry	Jan 2020
Exploratory IND Studies	Jan 2006
Nonclinical Safety Evaluation of the Immunotoxic Potential of Drugs and Biologics Guidance for Industry	Feb 2020
Rare Diseases: Natural History Studies for Drug Development Draft Guidance for Industry	Mar 2019
Physiologically Based Pharmacokinetic Analyses — Format and Content Guidance for Industry	Sep 2018
Biomarker Qualification: Evidentiary Framework	Dec 2018
Nonclinical Safety Evaluation of Reformulated Drug Products and Products Intended for Administration by an Alternate Route	Oct 2015
M3(R2) Nonclinical Safety Studies for the Conduct of Human Clinical Trials and Marketing Authorization for Pharmaceuticals: Questions and Answers	Mar 2013

7.5   Regulatory Pathways: 505(b)(1) and 505(b)(2)

505(b)(1) is the regulatory pathway used to obtain the approval of a new drug whose active ingredients have not previously been approved. This is the traditional New Drug Application (NDA) pathway.

505(b)(2) is the regulatory pathway used for drugs that contain similar active ingredients to a previously approved drug. This process involves a shorter drug development program and requires less resources than the 505(b)(1) regulatory pathway. It allows for new formulations, combination products, or routes of administration, for example.

Appendix

Chemical Nomenclature

General Nomenclature for Organic Compounds

General prefix for a carbon chain of any length: alk-.
General suffix for a functional group moiety: -yl.

Prefixes based on length of carbon chain:

C1: meth-	C4: but-	C7: hept-	C10: dec-
C2: Eth-	C5: Pent-	C8: Oct-	
C3: Prop-	C6: Hex-	C9: Non-	

Suffixes based on carbon saturation:

Single bond (saturated)	-ane
Double bond	-ene
Triple bond	-yne

Suffixes and prefixes for common functional groups.

Functional group	Suffix	Prefix
Acyl	-oyl	Acyl-
Aldehyde	-al	None
Alcohol	-ol	Hydroxyl-
Amide	-oic	None
Carboxylic acid	-oic acid	None
Carboxylic acid salt or ester	-oate	None
Ketone	-one	Keto- or oxo-
Nitrile	-nitrile	Cyano-

© Springer Nature Switzerland AG 2022
S. C. Khojasteh et al., *Discovery DMPK Quick Guide*,
https://doi.org/10.1007/978-3-031-10691-0

Prefixes for heteroatoms.

Element	Valence	Prefix
Nitrogen (N)	3	Aza-
Oxygen (O)	2	Oxa-
Sulfur (S)	2	Thia-
Phosphorous (P)	3	Phospha-

Common suffixes for nitrogen-containing and non-nitrogen-containing heterocycles.

Ring size	Saturated		Unsaturated	
	with N	without N	with N	without N
3	-iridine	-irane	-irine	-irene
4	-etidine	-etane	-ete	-ete
5	-olidine	-olane	-ole	-ole
6	-inine	-inane (−ane)	-ine	-ine

Note that if the ring contains some degree of unsaturation, the prefixes dihydro- or tetrahydro- are added accordingly.

Five-Membered Heterocyclic Rings

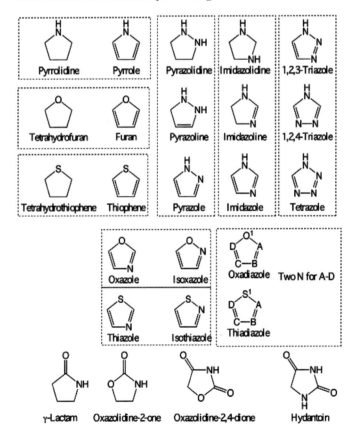

Six-Membered Heterocyclic Rings

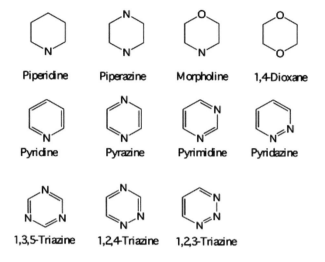

Piperidine   Piperazine   Morpholine   1,4-Dioxane

Pyridine   Pyrazine   Pyrimidine   Pyridazine

1,3,5-Triazine   1,2,4-Triazine   1,2,3-Triazine

Bicyclic Heterocycles

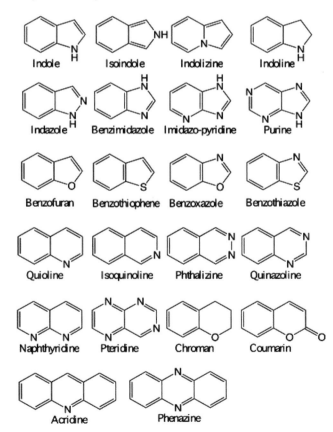

Indole   Isoindole   Indolizine   Indoline

Indazole   Benzimidazole   Imidazo-pyridine   Purine

Benzofuran   Benzothiophene   Benzoxazole   Benzothiazole

Quioline   Isoquinoline   Phthalizine   Quinazoline

Naphthyridine   Pteridine   Chroman   Coumarin

Acridine   Phenazine

Index

Printed in the United States
by Baker & Taylor Publisher Services